Healthy
Balance

In life *and*
In the Kitchen

Shannon Burrs

XULON PRESS

Xulon Press
2301 Lucien Way #415
Maitland, FL 32751
407.339.4217
www.xulonpress.com

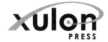

Spoon image used throughout book was designed by Pause08 and provided from Flaticon.com
Cover and lifestyle photos provided by Krista Brinkmeier Photography
Recipe photos provided by Shannon Burrs
Lifestyle photo setting taken at Four Winds Farm Fitchburg

Paperback ISBN-13: 978-1-6628-2115-8
Hard Cover ISBN-13: 978-1-6628-2116-5
Ebook ISBN-13: 978-1-6628-2117-2

A
Healthy
Balance

In life *and*
In the Kitchen

Recipe of the Day

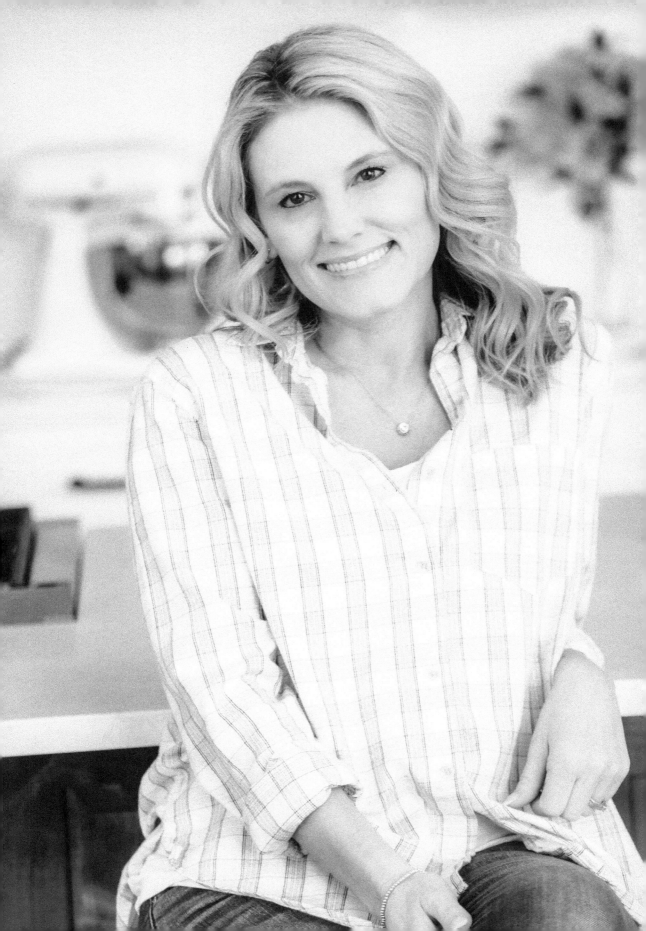

About the Author

⁓

SHANNON BURRS IS A WIFE AND MOTHER OF FOUR, AS WELL as a Wisconsin native and writer behind the blog of Faith.Food.Farm. Shannon has spent most of her professional life in dentistry and only recently started exploring the world of food photography and blogging. Shannon earned her master's degree in adult education and training from the University of Wisconsin Stout and currently works in dental operations. Outside of cooking and blogging, Shannon enjoys traveling, boating, and spending time with friends and family.

Married to a born and raised farmer— and a lover of animals herself, Shannon has discovered an appreciation for life on the farm. Recently the Burrs family made the decision to trade suburban life for country living and are in the process of building their own *farmette* to accommodate their horse and chickens, and love of gardening.

Find Shannon on Instagram @faith.food.farm to follow her journey of exploring all the joys that cooking and farm life have to offer.

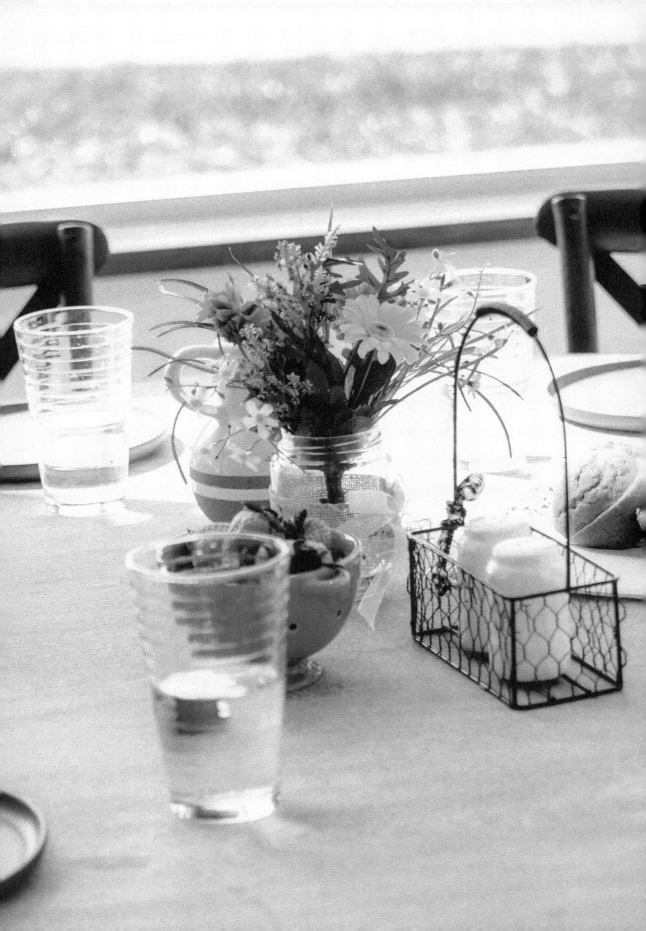

Welcome to My Kitchen

⁓

IF YOU HAD TOLD ME A PANDEMIC WOULD TAKE OVER THE world and change everything about life as we knew it in 2020, I would have never believed you. Most of us would agree; the last year and a half has sure been one for the books. Many people found themselves feeling rundown, overwhelmed, and ready for it to be over.

I too felt this way; that is until I decided it was time to get out of my rut and focus on the wellness of my mind and body. I aimed at eating healthier and being more mindful as I went about my days. I started sharing these thoughts and ideas with friends, and before I knew it, I was blogging. As I continued down this path, I discovered the versatility of recipes and began modifying them with healthy alternatives. Throughout this process, I came to realize there are more ways than one to make a good recipe. What tastes good to me may not taste good to everyone— the outcome depends on the recipient.

Perhaps I've spent too much time in the kitchen, but I have started looking at life through a similar lens. Life is made up of a series of moments. These moments, like ingredients, create the recipe of our life. Sometimes it's trial and error, but we can alter and improve them at any time to change the end result. A good life does not consist of one single ingredient, but many that include moments, people and experiences. Being mindful, present, and living with full intention allows us to make modifications when necessary and savor the moments that matter most.

I am forever grateful to the community of bloggers I've met along the way and those who have supported me on this journey. I thank God for placing this passion in my heart and for my beautiful family for inspiring me to be the best mom and wife I can be. Finally, I want to thank my parents for teaching me about compassion and sharing the joys of being in the kitchen.

This book is intended to be more than just a cookbook. The pages are meant for you to read, write on and refer back to whenever you need a positive reminder or delicious recipe. I'm glad you stopped by for a visit—let's get cooking!

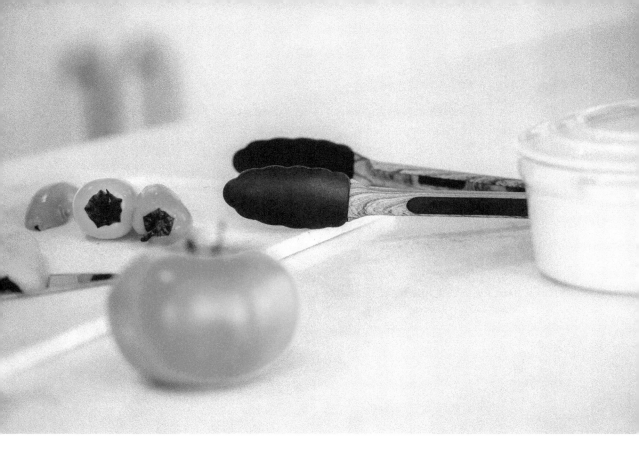

Clean Eating and Healthy Substitutes

"There are more ways than one to make a good recipe." – Shannon Burrs

A S SOMEONE WHO HAS TRIED A FEW DIET TRENDS, I'VE come up with my own idea of what healthy eating looks like for me. I have centered on the concept of balance. Maintaining a *healthy balance* allows me to live and be healthy without having the restrictions of a diet. Instead, I take everyday recipes that I like and love, and modify them just enough to eliminate some of the guilt.

As I began researching how to cook and eat cleaner, the most important lesson I learned was *how* to grocery shop. The pandemic forced me into a routine of online grocery shopping, which I later found to be a great way of staying disciplined in my choices. Making and sticking to a list of buying what I *need* versus what *sounds good* has made all the difference.

Another thing I learned was the importance of buying *fresh*. Once I have my cup-boards stocked with basic staple ingredients (such as those listed on the pages ahead), the majority of my weekly shopping consists of *fresh* foods such as produce, meats and dairy. Picture in your mind how a grocery store is designed. Generally speaking, fresh items are found along the outer edges of the store, while the aisles in the middle contain mostly processed or boxed foods. Think "outside the box" when you grocery shop—*think fresh*.

During the process of modifying and trying different recipes, I pulled together a list of healthy substitutions for commonly used ingredients. Throughout this book, you will see these and be able to incorporate them into the recipes I share.

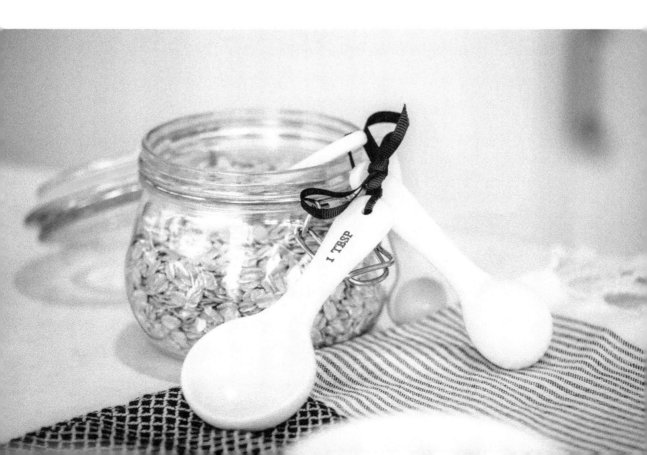

HEALTHY SUBSTITUTES

Swerve – Granular and confectioner sugar substitutes
Swerve Sweetener is made from natural ingredients that are sourced from the United States and France. With zero calories and zero net carbs, Swerve is certified non-GMO and non-glycemic, which means it does not raise your blood sugar. It is recommended to use this product in small amounts, as erythritol and oligosaccharides, the two main ingredients in Swerve, have been associated with digestive problems for some people.[1]

Monk fruit – Granulated sugar substitute
Monk fruit is derived from a small, green melon that contains natural sugars such as fructose and glucose. Despite its super-sweet taste, the body metabolizes monk fruit differently than it metabolizes table sugar. The same substance that gives monk fruit its sweetness is also the one that holds its anti-inflammatory properties, as an added benefit. There are currently no known adverse side effects of monk fruit, and it is "generally recognized as safe" by the Food and Drug Administration.[2]

Liquid aminos – Soy sauce substitute
Liquid aminos look and taste similar to soy sauce, adding a savory, salty flavor to meals without all the added sodium. Naturally vegan and gluten-free, liquid aminos also contain amino acids that are the building blocks of proteins.[3]

Almond flour – All-purpose flour substitute
Almond flour is gluten-free, low in carbs, and packed with nutrients such as vitamin E and magnesium. Generally speaking, almond flour may be better than conventional flours for blood sugar, as it has a low glycemic index.[4]

Coconut flour
Coconut flour is gluten-free and delivers 20 percent DV iron (plant-based), which has been linked to boosting energy, promoting weight loss, and reducing the growth of harmful bacteria. It is high in fiber and can help aid in digestion and keeping blood sugar low. Coconut flour is both denser and drier than other flour types, making it extremely absorbent.
For substitution purposes: **¼ cup of coconut flour = 1 cup all-purpose flour.**[5]

Coconut sugar – Natural sugar substitute
Unlike traditional table sugar, coconut sugar contains nutrients such as zinc, calcium, and potassium. It is healthier than refined sugar but is still high in calories and should be used sparingly.[6]

Honey – Natural sugar substitute
Honey contains trace amounts of vitamins and minerals as well as an abundance of antioxidants. Honey can be used as a sugar substitute in many recipes.[7]

Maple syrup – Natural sugar substitute
Maple syrup contains a decent amount of minerals and vitamins including calcium, potassium, iron and zinc as well as antioxidants. Maple syrup has a lower glycemic index than traditional sugar but can still raise blood sugar levels. Use sparingly as a sugar substitute in recipes.[8]

Applesauce – Natural sugar substitute – also used to substitute bananas, butter, and oil in some recipes.
Applesauce adds moisture and natural sweetness to many recipes. The ratio of substitution varies by recipe. In foods that do not need to be heated, applesauce can be equally substituted in side dishes, such as sweet potato casserole or baked beans. Applesauce adds both sweetness and flavor.[9]

Plain Greek yogurt – Sour cream substitute
Greek yogurt makes an excellent substitute for sour cream because it is lower in calories and fat while higher in protein. Greek yogurt is versatile and lasts longer than regular sour cream.[10]

Coconut oil – Butter substitute
Coconut oil has many health benefits that help maintain the liver, kidneys, skin, hair and other parts of the body. Coconut oil helps manage digestive distress as well as regulates blood sugar.[11]

Coconut milk – Heavy cream
Full-fat coconut milk is a great vegan, dairy-free substitute for heavy whipping cream.

Neufchatel cheese – Regular cream cheese
Neufchatel cheese has more protein and riboflavin, while less fat and cholesterol, than traditional cream cheese.[12]

Condiments – Ketchup, barbecue sauce, relish
Replacing condiments with no-sugar options is a great way of reducing your daily caloric intake.

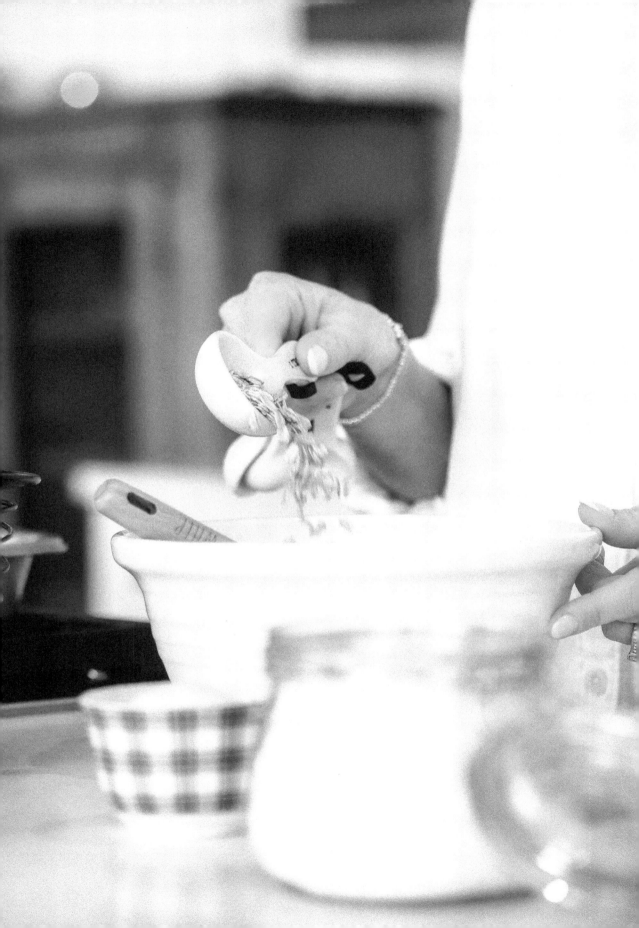

1

Purpose

"Certain things catch your eye but pursue only those that capture the heart."
– Ancient Indian Proverb[13]

THE INTERNET IS FILLED WITH MANY BLOGGERS—SO many that one could easily talk themselves out of continuing their work. But I remain faithful to my passion for inspiring and reminding others to look for the good in the world despite some of the chaos.

Cooking, and trying new recipes, is all part of the fun of blogging, but finding a bigger purpose in what I do is what pushes me to do more. A *purpose* consists of needs and values that drive us forward in life. Living intentionally allows us the opportunity to pursue our passion and purpose for life. Later in this book, you will read how my personal experiences have instilled certain passions in my heart. Cultivating positivity and promoting self-development are to name a couple that offer me a sense of purpose—for that reason, I wrote this book.

I believe we all have our own unique purpose and each of us will shine when we start living it. Searching inward and discovering what fulfills you will guide you toward discovering yours. I hope the messages will leave you feeling hopeful, mindful, and at peace as you go about your days and help drive you toward finding your own passion and purpose for life.

Challenge of the Day: **Take a quiet moment to write down something you are passionate about. Are you pursuing your purpose in life? If not, start by exploring all the things you love that make you happy. Form a goal from this list, and begin working toward fulfilling your own passion and purpose in life.**

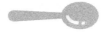

RECIPE OF THE DAY:

SUNSHINE SMOOTHIE

INGREDIENTS

½ cup plain vanilla Greek yogurt
1 cup frozen pineapple
1 cup low-sugar orange juice
1 frozen banana
1 cup ice

INSTRUCTIONS

Combine all ingredients together in a blender until smooth. Place in a glass and serve with fresh fruit.

Serves 1-2
Prep: 5 mins
Cook: none

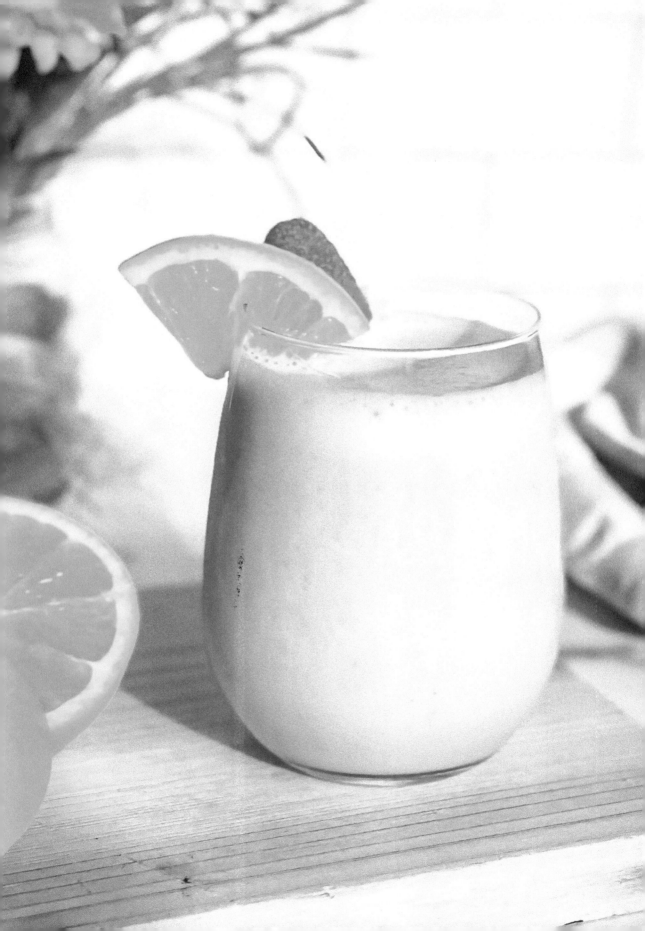

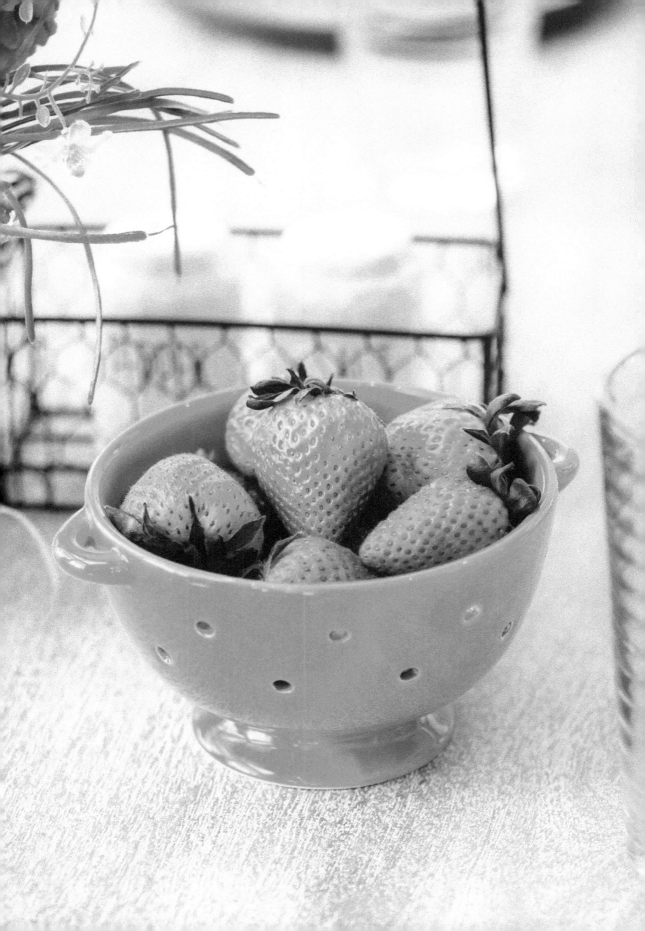

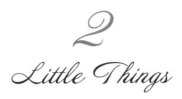

2
Little Things

*"Enjoy the little things, for one day you may look back
and realize they were the big things." –Robert Brault*

KENNY CHESNEY HAS A SONG CALLED "DON'T BLINK,"
where he speaks of all the little things in life—babies turning into adults almost
overnight, starting kindergarten one day, then suddenly out into the real world,
living carefree, then finding love and getting married. Having four kids of my own,
I know the words in this song all too well. I have watched our kids hit one mile-
stone after another like a whirlwind before my eyes—from learning to ride a bike
to driving a car, from graduating high school to moving into their first apartment.
As I drop them off at college one by one, my eyes fill with tears and my only hope
is that I leave their hearts and minds filled with many little things they can carry
throughout their lifetime.

Time is something that slips through our fingers. We always think we have more
of it, so we often bypass the "little things." Dinners around the table get replaced
with drive-thru meals eaten on our way to the next event. Family board games and
laughter are replaced with silence around the TV. Playing *I-Spy* in the car is replaced
with devices to occupy our minds until the destination is reached. There are so many
distractions available to interrupt our little things.

However, if you take a moment to ask someone in the later part of his or her life what
was most important, the person will, without a doubt, tell you it was the little things.

Challenge of the Day: **Go for a drive and find a dirt road or a field lined with
flowers. Take a moment to enjoy the beautiful blue sky and fresh air. To make
it even more memorable, do it with someone you love.**

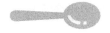

RECIPE OF THE DAY:
STRAWBERRY FIELDS SALAD

INGREDIENTS

1 bag (8 oz) mixed salad greens
1 cucumber, peeled and sliced thin
1 cup strawberries, sliced
½ cup blueberries
¼ cup candied pecans
¼ cup crumbled feta cheese
4 slices turkey deli meat, julienned
1 cup dried cranberries

DRESSING

¼ cup apple cider vinegar
3 tablespoons honey
3 tablespoons white sugar (Swerve)
2 teaspoons Dijon mustard
½ cup olive oil
Squeeze of fresh lemon

INSTRUCTIONS

Assemble salad and combine dressing ingredients to serve.

Serves 2-4
Prep: 15 mins
Cook: none

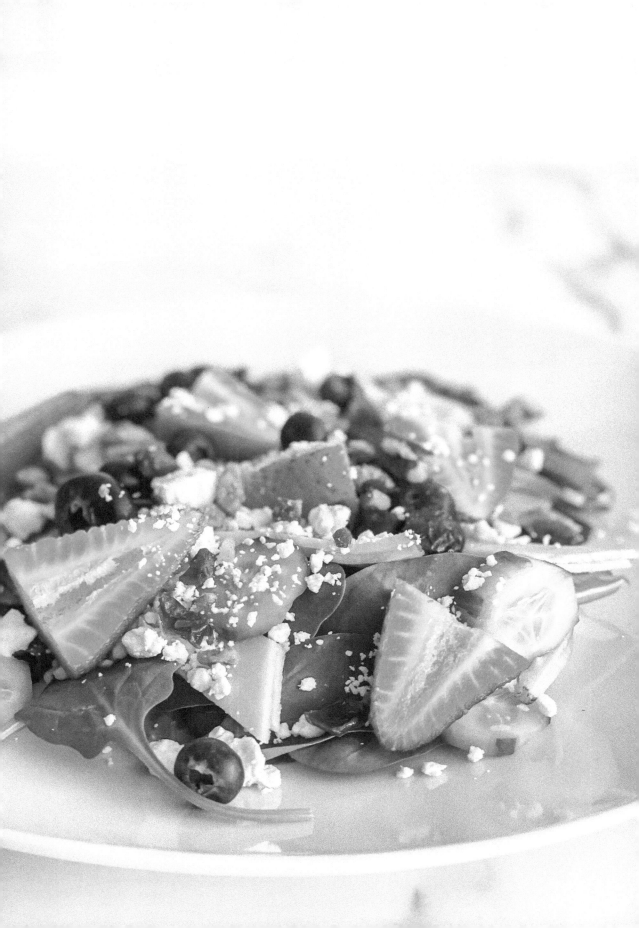

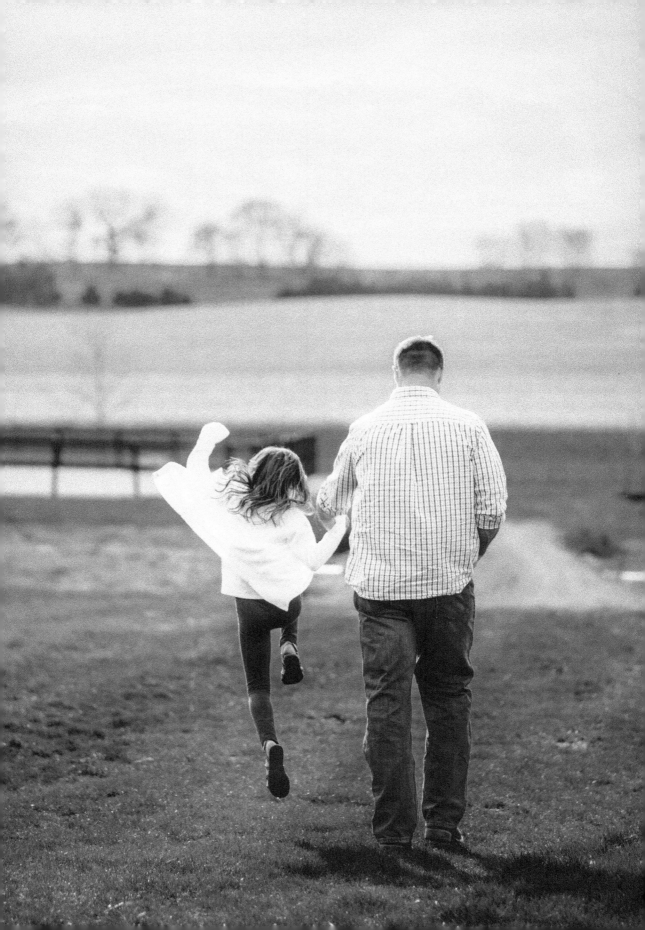

3

Simplicity

"The simple pleasures of life give us lasting satisfaction." – Avijeet Das

I GREW UP IN A SMALL SUBURBAN COMMUNITY WITH NEIGH-bors all around me; I couldn't fathom the idea of living any other way. I believed one day I would raise my kids the same, and until recently, that's just what I did. Ten years ago, I married my husband— a born-and-raised farmer. Over time, he planted a passion for farm life within me. It's not elegant or fancy; it's hard work and dedication, but above all—it takes you back to the basics.

The pandemic of 2020 really made me appreciate simplicity. Slowing down, growing a garden, spending quality time with the family: these are a few of the reasons we decided to sell our house and move out to the country. For me, slowing down requires serious effort and dedication. The constant need to be busy is always lurking around the corner. The truth is when I'm busy, I'm not present. When I live with full intention, I recognize areas in my life that need more attention and others that should be put aside. Slowing down and re-focusing my energy is what *simplicity* means for me.

Simplicity looks different for everyone. Of course, you do not need to sell everything and move out to the country to achieve this. You can still have nice things and live the life you want to live with full intention and mindfulness. Being able to balance life's busyness with all the little things that matter most can offer you wholeness and fulfillment. There are many ways people are finding simplicity. Spending more time in nature and dedicating quality family time are just to name a few. There isn't a right or wrong way of slowing down and living life a bit more simply. Each of us should decide what "simple" looks like for us and apply it.

Challenge of the Day: **Think of ways you could be living a simpler life. Of those, form a goal with the ones you are willing to make happen today.**

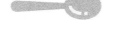

RECIPE OF THE DAY:
SIMPLE BREAKFAST SKILLET

INGREDIENTS

2 tablespoons olive oil
4 cups peeled, cooked and cubed sweet potatoes
2 tablespoons chili powder
2 teaspoons ground cumin
1 tablespoon lime zest
1 squeeze of lime juice
2 sweet bell peppers, sliced
1 small red onion, sliced
1 tablespoon chopped fresh cilantro
Eggs – cooked to preference
Salt and Pepper to taste

INSTRUCTIONS

Heat 1 tablespoon of olive oil in a large skillet over medium heat.
Add sweet potato, onions, peppers, chili powder, cumin, salt, pepper
and cilantro.
Cover and simmer for 8-10 minutes – stir frequently.
Remove potatoes and vegetables from pan and set aside.
Wipe pan clean. Add 1 tablespoon olive oil to skillet on medium heat. Cook
desired number of eggs to preference.
Serve with eggs cooked to preference.
Top with squeeze of lime juice and
zest.

Serves 2
Prep: 15 mins
Cook: 10 mins

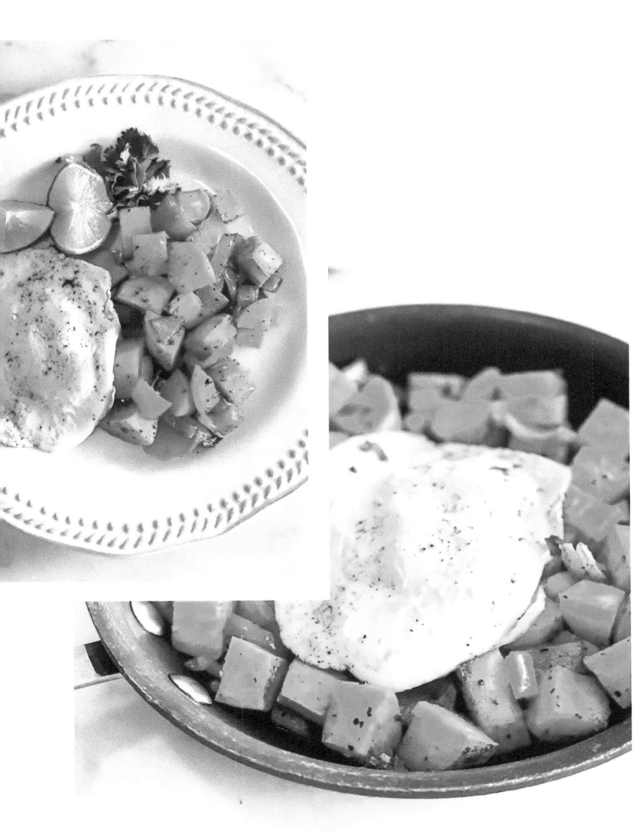

4
Comparison

"Comparison is the thief of joy." – Teddy Roosevelt

COMPARING OURSELVES TO OTHERS IS INEVITABLE WHEN the majority of human connection revolves around social media. How can we be satisfied with who we are and what we have when we are constantly looking at everyone else? We need to stop comparing.

I am least satisfied when I start comparing myself to others. Someone will always have more likes and followers than me on Instagram. Someone will always have things I can't afford. Someone will always be taller, skinnier, prettier, smarter, and have more friends than me. But no one will ever be me. I am uniquely *me* and no one else. I am on my own journey, and how I reach the finish line is mine and mine only. Comparison will only tarnish my experience getting there.

Humans were created to be different. Imagine a world where everyone was exactly the same: same look, same talent, same perspective. How boring would that be? How many discoveries and breakthroughs would never have happened if everyone were the same? Dare to be different. Think of the most innovative leaders from history: Albert Einstein, Sir Isaac Newton, Thomas Edison. Those are just a few of the many brilliant minds who have made an impact on the world as we know it.

You weren't created as a unique individual just so you could conform to a mold someone else came from. We should all add our own flavor to the mix of this life.

Challenge of the Day: **Take a moment to reflect on what makes you, YOU. What are your unique talents? Recognize that being different is a gift. Embrace what makes you stand out from the crowd. There's only one YOU.**

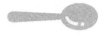

RECIPE OF THE DAY:

BERRY YOGURT PARFAIT

INGREDIENTS

1 cup plain or vanilla Greek yogurt
1 cup fresh berries of choice (strawberries, blueberries, raspberries)
⅓ cup granola
2 tablespoons low-sugar fruit preserves
½ lemon for zest and juice.

INSTRUCTIONS

In a glass jar, layer bottom with fruit preserves.
Place yogurt over top. followed by fresh fruit.
Add granola. Repeat layers.
Add lemon zest over top with a squeeze of juice.

Serves 1-2
Prep: 20 mins
Cook: none

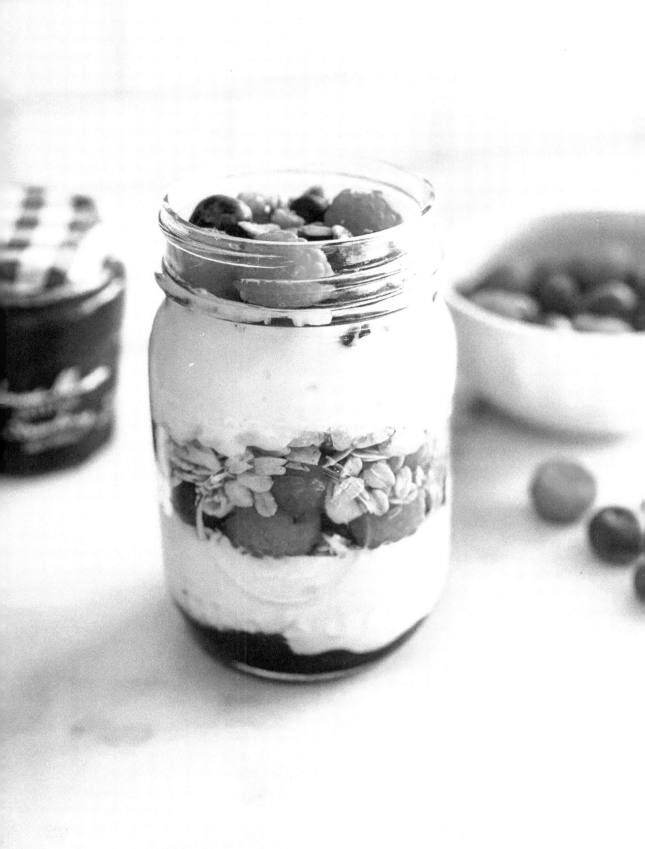

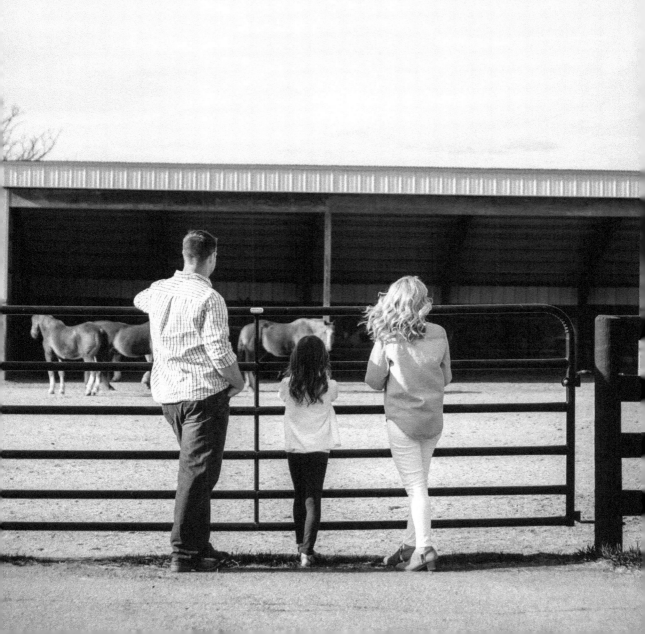

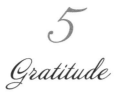

5
Gratitude

"Gratitude helps us see what is there instead of what isn't." – Annette Bridges

I AM SURE EACH OF US COULD WRITE DOWN AT LEAST TEN things we wish we had more of or places we could go. There's always a desire to want more. However, when we practice gratitude, we become mindful of things we already have.

Earlier this year, I invited my followers on Instagram to join me in a thirty-day gratitude challenge. I wasn't sure if anyone would take part in it, but I was amazed by the response and how many people reached out and participated. When I think about all the reasons to be grateful, I suddenly want and need less. For every "want," I can always offset it with something I already have.

Research has linked gratitude with enhancing the immune system, lowering blood pressure, increasing positive emotions, and reducing loneliness and isolation.[14] There are so many things around us, big and small, that we can be grateful for. Family dinners...coffee with friends...the laughter of children...just to name a few. Focusing on these good things in our lives is the best way to adapt an attitude of gratitude.

Challenge of the Day: **Find something or someone in your life to be grateful for and show your appreciation. Take time to phone a friend, write a letter, paint a picture, or bake a family recipe. The opportunities are endless when you find gratitude.**

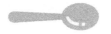

RECIPE OF THE DAY:

SIGNATURE CHILI

INGREDIENTS

1 pound lean ground turkey or beef
1 tablespoon olive oil
1 can mild chili beans, do not drain
2 cans petite diced tomatoes, do not drain
1 packet low-sodium McCormick chili seasoning
1 green pepper, finely diced
1 yellow onion, finely diced
2 tablespoons minced garlic
2 cups low-sodium tomato juice
½ teaspoon Cajun seasoning
1 tablespoon pure maple syrup
Optional Toppings: Plain Greek yogurt, shredded cheddar cheese, parsley

INSTRUCTIONS

Heat a large skillet with olive oil. Add onion, garlic, and green pepper. Cook until soft and onion is translucent. Add ground turkey or beef to skillet and cook until brown.
Drain excess grease.
In a large stock or crock pot, place meat mixture. Add remaining ingredients.
Slow cooker: Cook on high 4 hours or low 6-8 hours.
Stovetop: Bring to a boil and reduce heat to low. Cover and allow to simmer for 20-30 minutes, stirring occasionally.

Serves 4
Prep: 20 mins
Cook: 30 mins

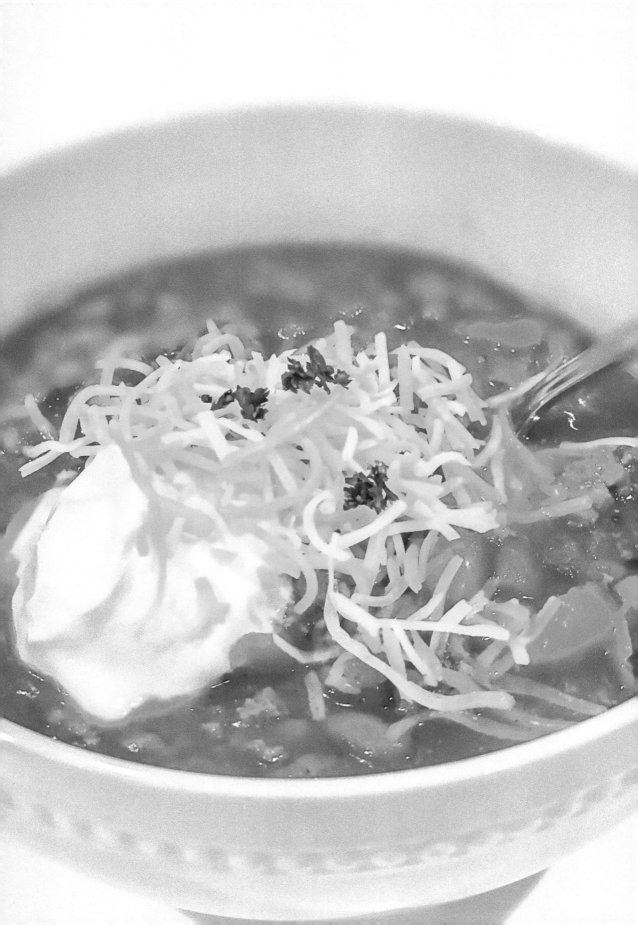

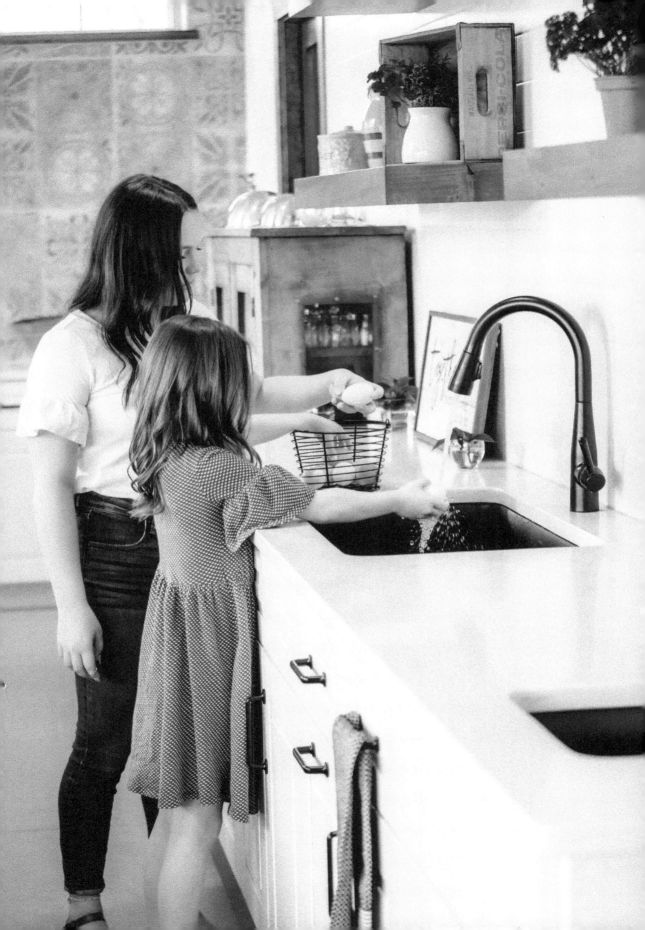

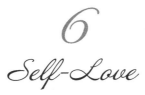

6

Self-Love

"Love yourself first and everything falls in line.
You really have to love yourself to get anything done in the world." – Lucille Ball

NOTHING FEELS BETTER THAN LOOKING AT YOURSELF IN the mirror and feeling good about the person looking back. Unfortunately, for most of us, the mirror is a place where every little flaw is amplified, almost as if we've highlighted everything we don't like about ourselves. We find a new blemish or wrinkle, our jeans look tighter, our hair is a mess and before you know it, we've picked ourselves apart.

Self-love is valuing and appreciating ourselves for who we are without apology. I am just as guilty as anyone reading this, and have plenty of work to do in this area. Like you, I doubt and second-guess myself for fear of how others might perceive me.

Negative thoughts like these cause unnecessary anxiety and prevent us from being our true selves. The truth is, if we appreciate and value our own thoughts and opinions, it shouldn't matter what others think. Easier said than done. Living and loving ourselves the way we deserve takes honest hard work, and it is likely the most important job we'll ever have.

Challenge of the Day: **Treat yourself right today. Do something you normally wouldn't do. Go to your favorite restaurant, treat yourself to a day of relaxation. Focus on loving yourself today.**

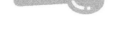

RECIPE OF THE DAY:

DRAGON FRUIT SMOOTHIE

INGREDIENTS

1 cup frozen dragon fruit chunks
¾ cup frozen strawberries
1 tablespoon lime juice
1 tablespoon honey
¼ teaspoon salt
¼ cup no-sugar cranberry juice
1 teaspoon ginger paste

INSTRUCTIONS

Combine all ingredients together in a blender until smooth.

Serves 1-2
Prep: 5 mins
Cook: none

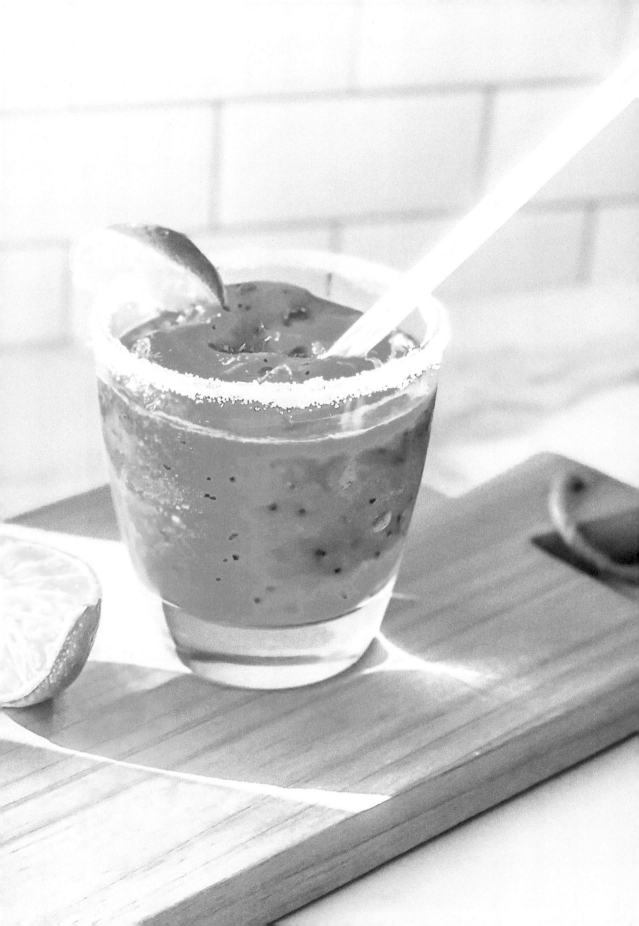

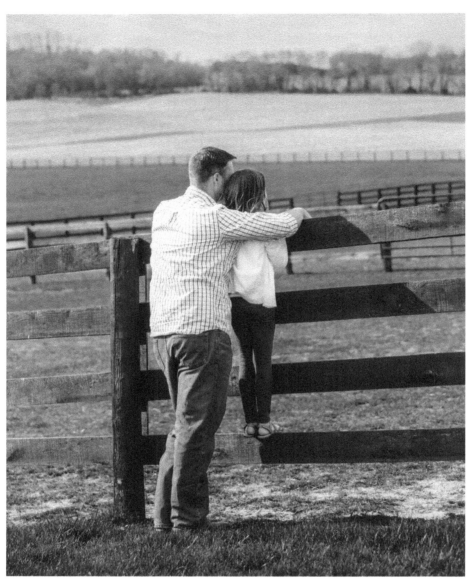

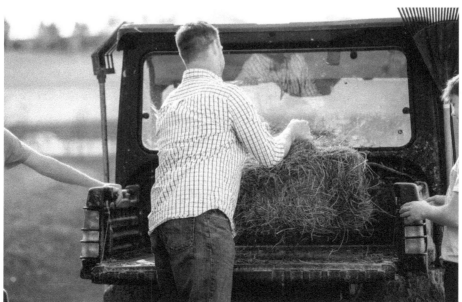

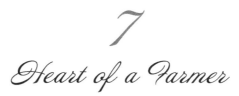

7

Heart of a Farmer

"The farmer has to be an optimist or he wouldn't still be a farmer." – Will Rogers

I've SEEN FIRST-HAND THE CHALLENGES THAT FARMERS can face in the work they do: droughts, floods, and climate change, just to name a few. However, despite these things, they go into each new season with an open and optimistic mind. Many of us could learn from this *keep on keeping on* attitude that farmers live by. Every day, in every situation, we have the choice to give up or stay on track and push through our challenges. Just as a farmer's dedication can determine the outcome of his crop, our dedication can determine the outcome of what we reap in our lives.

So many things a farmer does is out of their control—mother nature and fluctuating markets are just to name two. But if you ask any farmer, there is nothing more rewarding than planting a crop and watching the fruits of their labor come to completion. Farming is one of the few jobs where one can witness God's creation and continue what He started. In the end, farmers take pride in everything they do.

Hefty goals cannot be achieved if we throw in the towel right before the finish line. By exercising all the other things talked about in this book, *keep on keeping on* can become an attitude we live by as well. When we practice gratitude, pursue our passions, and learn to appreciate the little things in life, we will find ourselves more willing to stay the course.

Challenge of the Day: **Be a farmer at heart. This week, try to find the positive in every situation instead of focusing on the negative. Keep on keeping on!**

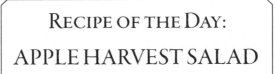

RECIPE OF THE DAY:

APPLE HARVEST SALAD

INGREDIENTS

1 bag (8 oz) mixed salad greens
2 cups cooked and diced chicken
¾ cup seedless grapes, diced in half
1 apple – cored, peeled, and thinly sliced
½ cup slivered almonds

DRESSING

¼ cup low-fat mayo
¼ cup plain Greek yogurt
1 tablespoon honey
1 tablespoon lemon juice
1 tablespoon fresh basil, finely chopped
½ teaspoon salt

INSTRUCTIONS

Combine chicken, apple, and grapes in a medium bowl, along with slivered almonds.
Combine mayo, yogurt, lemon juice, honey, basil, and salt in a small bowl.
Toss salad with dressing and serve.

Serves 2-3
Prep: 15 mins
Cook: none

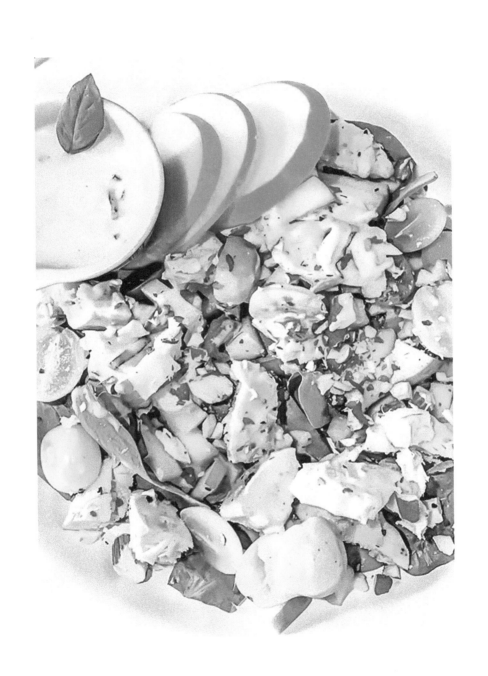

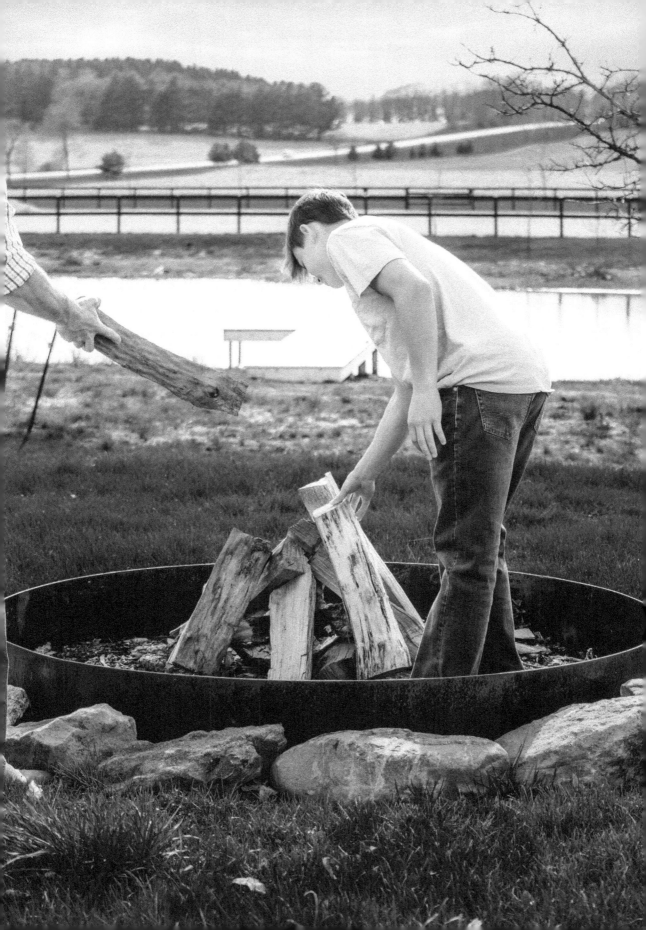

8

Fear

"Too many of us are not living our dreams because we are living our fears."
– Les Brown

FEAR IS A HEALTHY EMOTION; IT KEEPS US SAFE BY alerting us to danger. However, when we allow fear to be the driver of our lives, we give it too much power. When this happens, it can cripple and prevent us from doing something we were meant to do.

Whether it is fear of failure or fear of rejection, *fear is immobilizing*. It stops us dead in our tracks even when we have the means to move forward. If we allow fear to hold us back, we will likely miss some of the greatest opportunities in our lives.

Living intentionally helps us recognize exactly what drives the decisions we make.

Don't allow fear to prevent you from reaching your goals or chasing your dreams. If I did, you wouldn't be reading this book.

Challenge of the Day: **Take a moment to reflect on a time when fear stopped you from doing something. Would you go back and do it over if you could?**

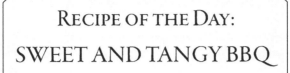

RECIPE OF THE DAY:

SWEET AND TANGY BBQ

INGREDIENTS

1 pound lean ground beef or turkey
½ yellow onion, finely diced
4 tablespoons finely chopped pickle
1 cup no-sugar ketchup
3 teaspoons sweet and tangy mustard
3 teaspoons pure maple syrup
½ teaspoon chili powder
Salt and pepper to taste
Romaine or butter lettuce leaves
Finely shredded cheddar cheese

INSTRUCTIONS

In a large skillet, brown ground turkey or beef with diced onion. Season with chili powder, salt, and pepper. In a small bowl, combine ketchup, mustard, syrup, and pickle. Pour over meat; simmer uncovered 5 mins. Spoon meat mixture over lettuce or bread of choice and top with shredded cheese.

Serves 4
Prep: 10 mins
Cook: 30 mins

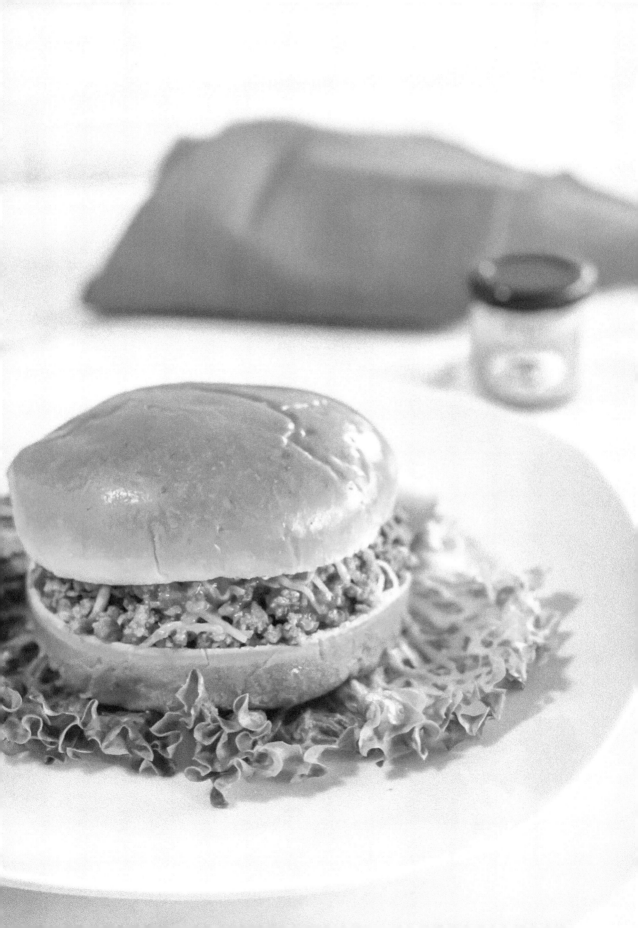

9
Confidence

*"The most common way people give up their power is
by thinking they don't have any." – Alice Walker*

W E PREVIOUSLY DISCUSSED HOW FEAR CAN HOLD YOU
back from following your dreams. Now let's talk about the way for you to
reach them—believe you can! Fear's ugly twin is self-doubt. Self-doubt overtakes
our minds and amplifies every failure. Anytime we try to move forward, self-doubt
is often right there to remind us of all the times we tried before and failed.

If you bake a batch of cookies and every single one turns out bad, you'll likely take
time to evaluate what went wrong. Did you miss an ingredient? Was there a step out
of turn? You don't just give up on baking cookies forever. We have to do the same
with our lives. Why did we fail that time? Did we charge forward without a plan?
Were we too impatient? Did we go at it alone when it should have been a team effort?

Mankind is capable of amazing things—this includes you! Amazing things can be
accomplished in and through our lives, but we have to believe in ourselves. We have
to become our own cheerleaders, recognizing and utilizing our abilities to their
fullest without doubt.

Challenge of the Day: **Is there an area in your life where you lack confidence?
Take a moment to reflect on why. Have you tried before and failed? Re-evaluate
and consider trying it again with a new approach.**

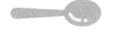

RECIPE OF THE DAY:
INSTANT POT CHICKEN CHILI

INGREDIENTS

1 yellow onion, diced
2 tablespoons minced garlic
2 (15 oz) cans Navy or Great
Northern White beans, drained
and rinsed
1 can white Shoepeg corn
2 cups low-sodium chicken broth
1 can (4 oz) diced green chiles
1 ½ teaspoons chili powder
1 teaspoon cumin

1 teaspoon oregano
2 chicken breasts, boneless
and skinless
Small bunch of cilantro,
finely chopped
½ cup plain Greek yogurt
2 oz Neufchatel cheese
½ lime, juiced
Salt and Pepper to taste

INSTRUCTIONS

Place all ingredients in pot except for yogurt, Neufchatel cheese and cilantro.
Close the lid.
Pressure cook on HIGH for 20 minutes.
Allow pressure to release.
Remove chicken and shred with a fork.
Return chicken to the pot, along with cilantro, yogurt, Neufchatel cheese, and
lime juice.
Stir well and serve.
Optional toppings: Serve with tortilla chips, Monterey Jack cheese, black
olives, avocados, plain yogurt, corn, and diced tomatoes.

Serves 4-6
Prep: 15 mins
Cook: 20 mins

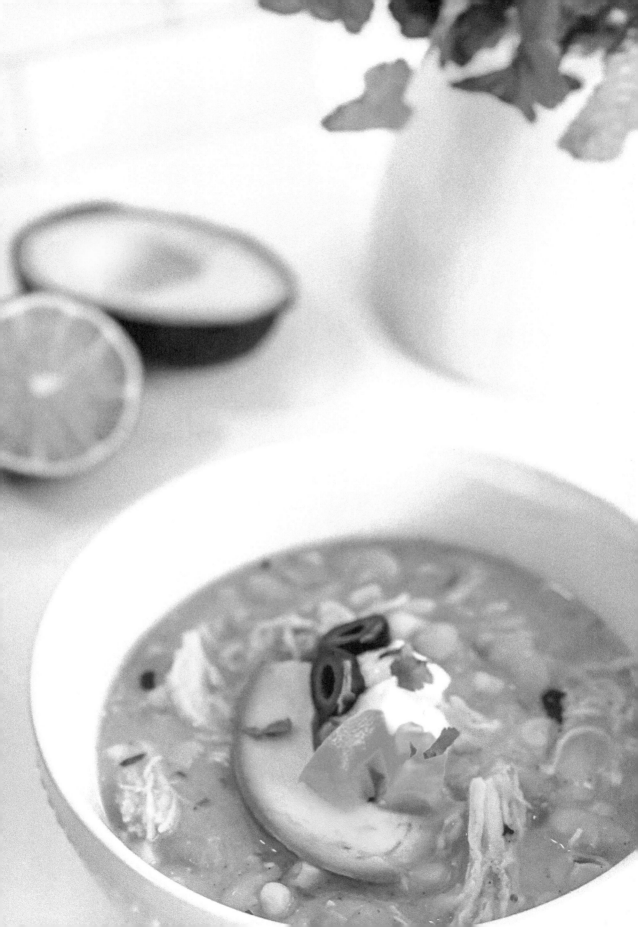

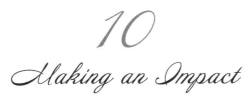

10

Making an Impact

"Life is about making an impact, not making an income." – Kevin Kruse

OFTENTIMES, WE FOCUS ON MATERIALISTIC THINGS AND forget there are small gestures with little to no cost that can make the biggest difference to others. Baking someone cookies, writing someone a letter, a friendly nod: these are all so simple and yet can leave such an impact on the heart of the recipient.

For myself, blogging certainly falls into this category. I can assure you that most bloggers do it for passion, and not to get anything back in return. There is a lot of hard work and time that goes into each and every post. Blogging is fun, but with it comes a fair amount of pressure. Yet when I receive a message from someone saying they were moved or impacted by a post I shared, I remember exactly why I do it.

The impact we have on others, big or small, is what counts. Maybe one of my readers will walk away with a new recipe and another will walk away encouraged to face another day. All I know is, no matter who the recipient is, I'm happy to be doing my part in making an impact.

Challenge of the Day: **Pay it forward! Find someone you can help today— something as simple as holding a door for someone, letting a car in front of you, or a passing smile—make an impact today.**

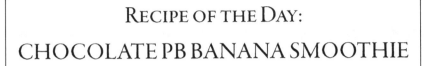

RECIPE OF THE DAY:

CHOCOLATE PB BANANA SMOOTHIE

INGREDIENTS

¼ cup natural creamy peanut butter
2 bananas, frozen
½ cup unsweetened almond milk
½ cup vanilla Greek yogurt
2 tablespoons cocoa powder
¾ cup ice

INSTRUCTIONS

Combine all ingredients together in a blender until smooth.

Serves 1-2
Prep: 5 mins
Cook: none

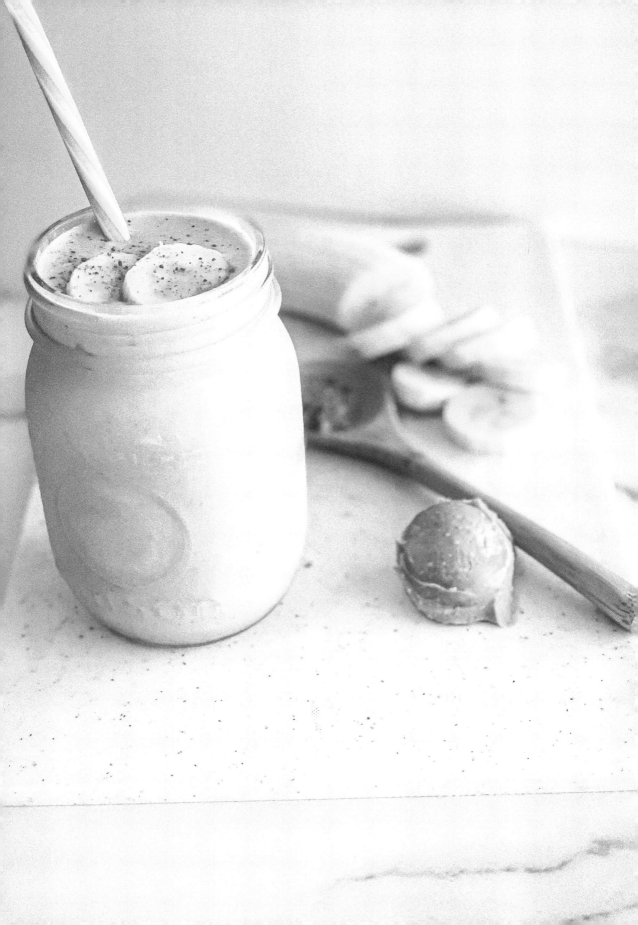

11
Don't Be a Crab

*"If people are doubting how far you can go,
go so far that you can't hear them anymore." –Michele Ruiz*

RECENTLY, I CAME ACROSS AN ARTICLE BY A FELLOW blogger, Sam Woolfe, about something called the Crab Mentality.[15] To sum up the article, when you put a bunch of crabs in a bucket, they begin clawing at each other and pulling each other down. As Woolfe says, *"...rather than let any crab survive or work together to escape, the crabs opt for a collective demise."*

Oftentimes, people are not much different from crabs in a bucket. How many times have you seen someone pull or put another person down because the person was jealous or envious of the other person getting "higher in the bucket"? Rather than encourage and be grateful for that person, they allow jealousy to get the best of them. At work, at home, or even in your own circle of friends this can happen. How much further would we get in life if we operated more like geese and less like crabs.

Canadian geese work together. They fly together in a V-formation, which requires a lot of effort from the goose at the tip of the V and less effort from those in the back. Geese understand the hardship it takes to be a leader within the flock. So, instead of fighting the goose who is at the front, they rotate within the formation. They take turns being leaders within their community. Another thing geese practice is *"no goose left behind."* If a goose is injured along the journey, another goose will stay with the injured goose and not leave until it recovers or dies.[16]

We cannot control the actions of others; however, we can decide if we will allow their negativity to change and control us. Eventually we must decide who makes us feel good and who doesn't. We have a choice to stay in those relationships or move on. Will we allow others to pull us back into the bucket, or will we push them to take a turn at the front of the flock?

Challenge of the Day: **Write down a situation when you experienced a negative encounter with a crab. How did that situation make you feel?**

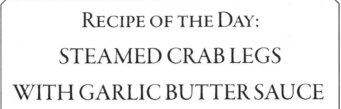

RECIPE OF THE DAY:
STEAMED CRAB LEGS
WITH GARLIC BUTTER SAUCE

INGREDIENTS

1 pound snow crab clusters, thawed
½ cup butter
1 teaspoon minced garlic
1 teaspoon dried parsley
1 lemon
¼ teaspoon salt

INSTRUCTIONS

Place thawed crab legs in a steamer basket in a large stock pot.
Add water and bring to a boil. Cover and steam 5-6 minutes or until heated through. Do not overcook.
Prepare garlic butter sauce: Combine melted butter, garlic, parsley, salt, and a fresh squeeze of lemon.
Serve immediately.

Serves 2
Prep: 10 mins
Cook: 10 mins

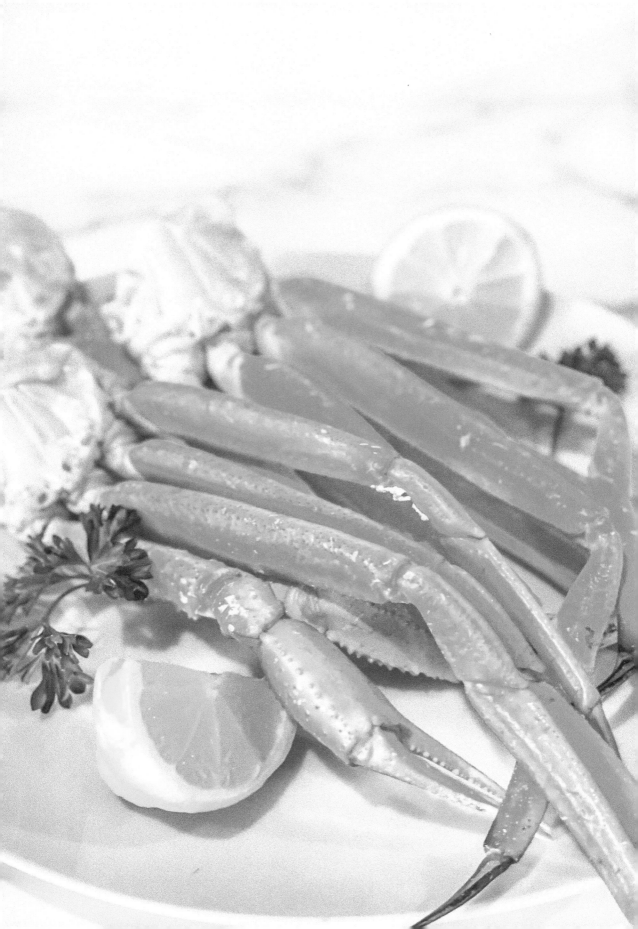

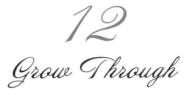

12
Grow Through

"You grow through—what you go through." – Tyrese Gibson

JUST LIKE YOU, I HAVE FACED MANY CHALLENGES. MY strength has been tested and at times it would have been a whole lot easier to wave a white flag of defeat. However, I found that in some of my darkest moments were the times I grew the most.

When things are going smooth, we don't have to stop and think too much about them. Like being on autopilot drifting through the air, you don't have a care in the world because everything is smooth and easy. But when struggles arise, it's time to be alert and ready to go. Pilots cannot coast through the air when storms arise or when conditions turn less than favorable. In those moments, they have to navigate through the difficult situations.

You are not the only person who goes through *stuff*. When we view other people's lives through filters on social media, everything looks too good to be true— that's probably because it is! Even I tend to share the happiest moments of my life with my readers. I do this intentionally, so people will leave feeling positive and uplifted from what they've just read. This does not mean that I live a life of perfection. Hopefully you have been able to see throughout the chapters in this book that just like you, I need reminders to slow down, enjoy the little things and be more confident. I can assure you that everybody experiences hard times. I've lived the pain of divorce, the death of my father, and the everyday petty nuisances that rise up here and there. No one is exempt!

In moments of struggle, we have the choice to be alert and navigate our way through— or—sit back, drifting on autopilot as chaos swirls around us. If a pilot did the latter of the two, what do you suppose would happen to the plane?

Challenge of the Day: **What is something you have been struggling with in your life recently? Are you on autopilot? Or, are you alert and navigating your way out through it?**

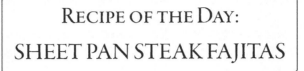

Recipe of the Day:

Sheet Pan Steak Fajitas

INGREDIENTS —————————————

1-2 steaks of choice (sirloin or round)
2 tablespoons olive oil, divided
1 yellow onion, thinly sliced
1 yellow bell pepper, thinly sliced
1 red bell pepper, thinly sliced
½ tablespoon low-sodium soy sauce (liquid aminos)
1 package of low-carb flour tortillas
2 tablespoons taco/fajita seasoning packet

INSTRUCTIONS —————————————

Preheat oven to 450 degrees.
Marinate steak: In a large plastic Ziplock© bag, combine 1 tablespoon olive oil, soy sauce, lime juice, and 1 tablespoon of seasoning mixture. Set aside.
Slice peppers and onions, and place in a bowl with remaining oil and seasoning mixture.
Toss to coat. On a lightly sprayed cookie sheet, arrange peppers and onions around outer edges. Add marinated steak to the center of the cookie sheet.
Cook at 450 degrees for 12-15 minutes—broil for an additional 2 minutes to crisp outer edges.
Let steak rest for 10 minutes, then slice against the grain.
Serve with warm tortillas and desired toppings.
Optional toppings: lettuce, tomatoes, shredded cheese, plain Greek yogurt, and diced avocado.

Serves 3-4
Prep: 20 mins
Cook: 30 mins

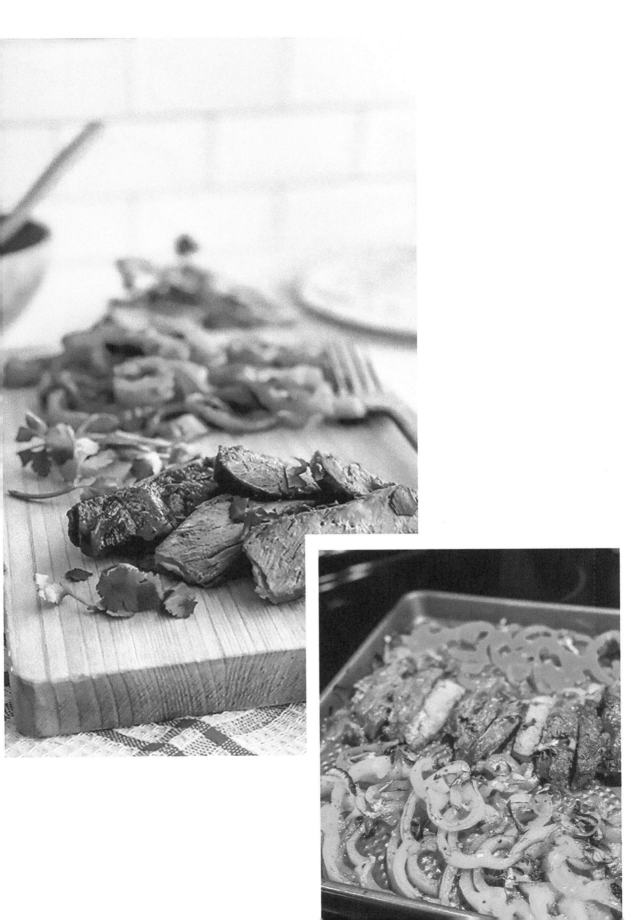

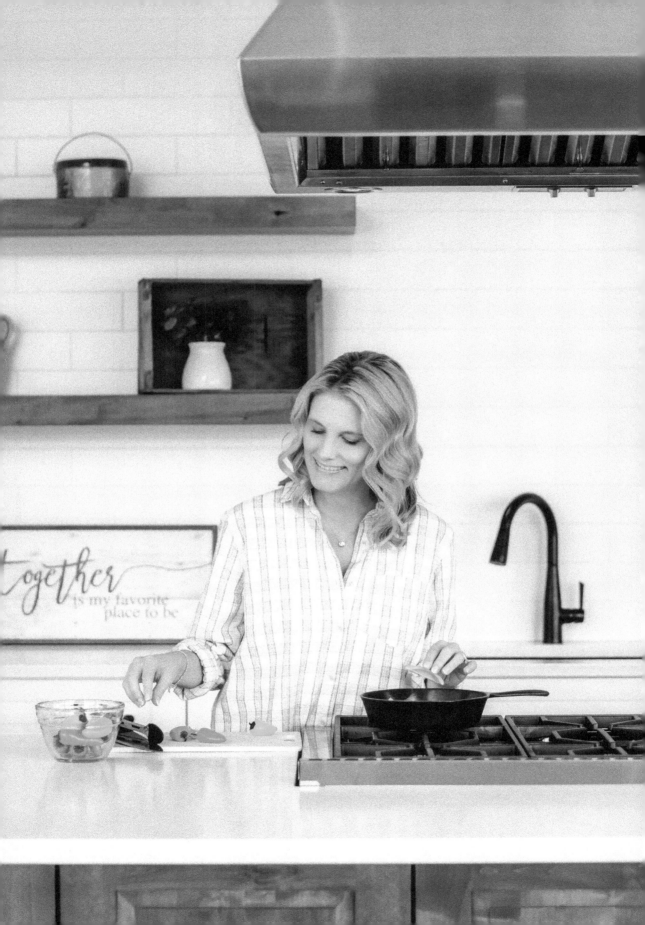

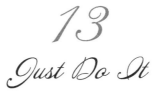

13
Just Do It

"Some people want it to happen, some wish it would happen, others make it happen." –Michael Jordan

WHEN WE DO NOTHING, NOTHING HAPPENS. BUT WHEN we do something, something happens. Sounds obvious, I know. The point is that the world is full of choices. Don't be *just* a talker or *just* a thinker; be a doer! Oftentimes, we find ourselves frustrated with various things in our lives—the cluttered closet, the messy drawers, the unfinished projects. All the while, we fail to admit we are the only ones who have the power to change these things.

It's time to prioritize what matters. If the closet is cluttered, clean it. If the drawers are messy, organize them. How much better will we feel once we have accomplished these tasks one at a time? It is time we stop regretting the things that WE have decided not to do.

When we prioritize what matters to us in life, we receive a reward like no other. Big or small, all accomplishments feel good. Just because something may seem insignificant compared to other things, it doesn't make it less important.

The state of our laundry, dirty dishes, or unfinished projects might not affect anyone else, but if they matter enough to bother us, we should do something about them.

Challenge of the Day: **Make it happen today. Find something you have been putting off and Just do it—today.**

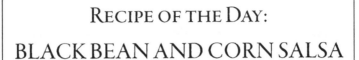

RECIPE OF THE DAY:

BLACK BEAN AND CORN SALSA

INGREDIENTS

1 (15 oz) can white shoepeg corn
1 (15 oz) can black beans, drained and rinsed
1 (14 .5 oz) can Italian-style petite diced tomatoes, drained
1 bunch finely chopped cilantro
1/2 cup chopped red onion
1 yellow bell pepper, seeded and chopped
¼ cup fresh lime juice
1 tablespoon olive oil or to taste
Salt and pepper to taste

INSTRUCTIONS

In a medium bowl combine corn, black beans, tomatoes, cilantro, red onion and bell pepper.
Stir in lime juice and drizzle with olive oil to serve.

Serve with tortilla chips

Serves 2-4
Prep: 15 min
Cook: none

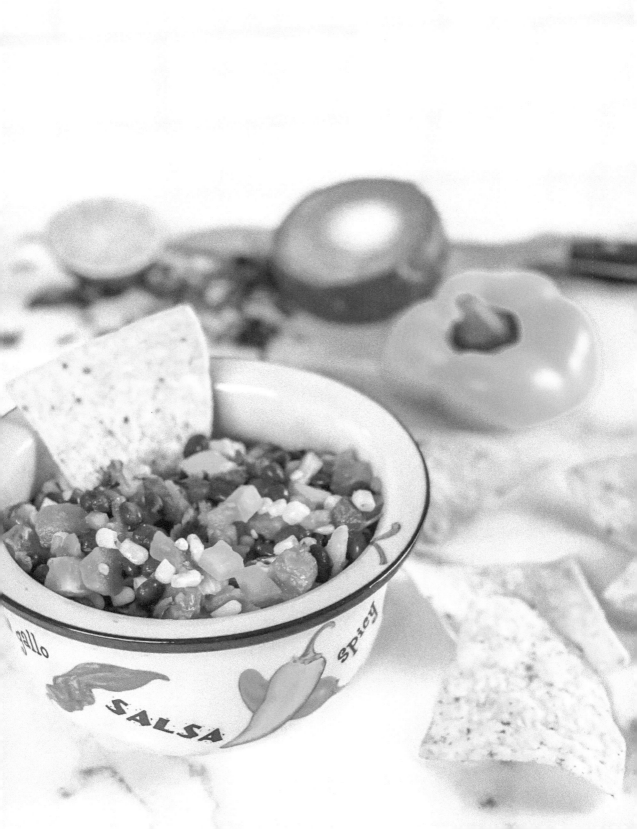

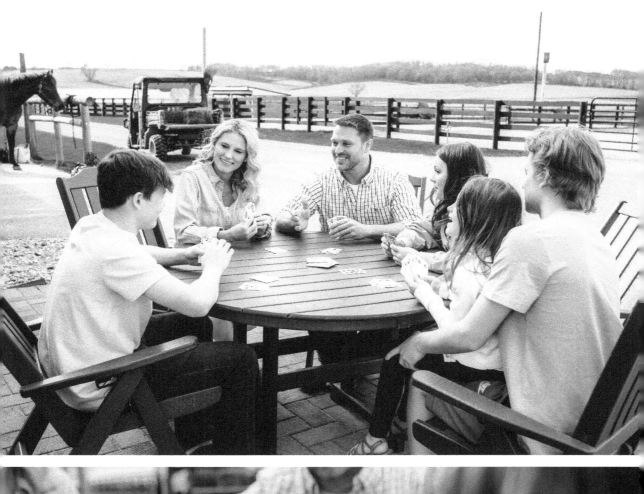
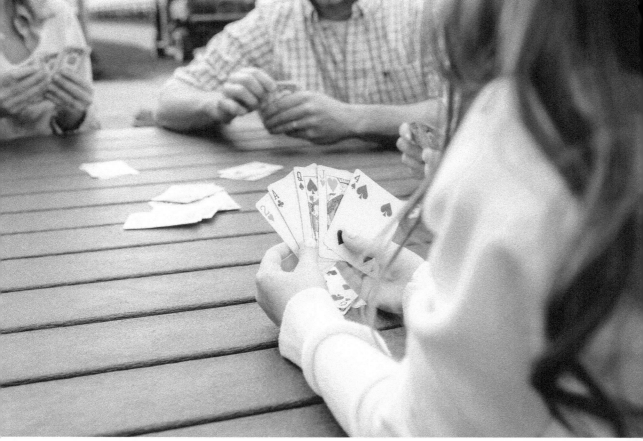

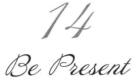

14

Be Present

"Your time is limited, so don't waste it living someone else's life." – Steve Jobs

I WAS IN EIGHTH GRADE WHEN MY DAD PASSED AWAY. AT the age of thirteen, I learned how short life could be. Now that I am older and have a family of my own, I think about all the things my dad never got to experience: weddings, graduations, grandchildren, and many other precious moments.

Life is short. We don't get to decide when our time is up, but we *do* get to decide what we do with the time we have.

It's easy to find ourselves separated from the moment. How many times have you caught yourself scrolling through your phone, only to find that minutes or hours have passed? It's easy to do, and you're not alone. Sometimes we take for granted the time we have here in this world without even knowing it. Since the start of the pandemic, I have found myself more attached than ever to my phone. I try minimizing this behavior by setting aside *no-screen* time and placing my phone in a separate room so I don't feel tempted to pick it up. All of these things are good practices but take a conscious effort.

Ten or twenty years from now, we won't remember the mindless moments spent on our phones, but we will remember a new activity or tradition we started with our families. Living in the present and enjoying each moment is not something that comes naturally. It is something that requires us to be mindful and purposeful. It takes hard work and dedication, but it will be well worth it in the end.

Challenge of the Day: **Set aside one whole day without social media. Take the time you would normally spend scrolling and spend it with those you love.**

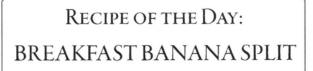

RECIPE OF THE DAY:

BREAKFAST BANANA SPLIT

INGREDIENTS

1 banana, cut in half lengthwise
½ cup Greek yogurt – flavor of choice
1 tablespoon almond milk
¼ cup granola
1 cup fresh berries of choice
1-2 tablespoons melted peanut butter or PB powder, prepared as directed

INSTRUCTIONS

Peel banana and cut in half lengthwise, and place on a plate.
Mix almond milk and yogurt to thin and pour over bananas.
Spread berries and granola over yogurt, and drizzle prepared peanut butter over bananas.

Serves 1-2
Prep: 15 mins
Cook: none

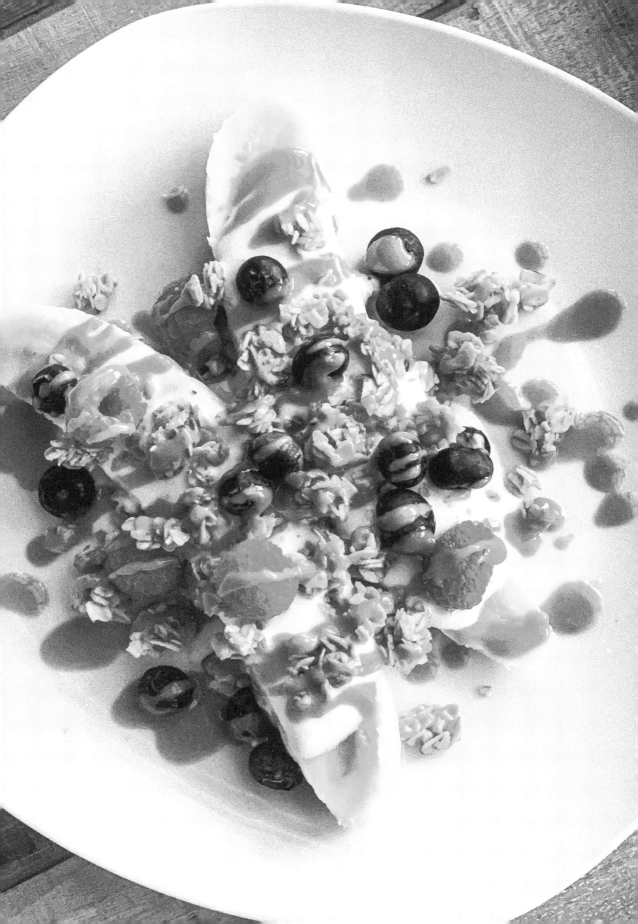

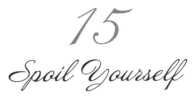

15
Spoil Yourself

"Sometimes we just need to take a little time for ourselves." – Unknown

WE TALKED ABOUT HOW LIFE IS SHORT AND THE IMPORTANCE of soaking up every possible moment we can with our loved ones, but all too often, we forget about ourselves. Adulting is hard. Whether you are a college kid experiencing life outside the home or a parent raising kids of your own, having responsibilities and being an adult can just sometimes be hard.

On top of that, we're often told not to be selfish. With this is mind, how do we decipher between caring for ourselves and being selfish? I'm not sure if it is the same for men, but I know most women can relate to this when it comes to buying a new outfit or treating themselves to a day at the salon. Why do we sometimes feel guilty for spending a little extra time and money on ourselves? If it makes us feel good, why not?

The same can be true of our mental state of being. Nobody can see inside our mind; they do not know when we are overworked or overwhelmed, which is why it is even more important for us to be in tune with our own well-being. We are the only ones who can truly take care of ourselves because only we know when we have hit our limit. We must listen to what our minds and bodies are telling us—do we need a nap, a vacation, some sunlight?

Take time for yourself. Yes, the dishes need washing, the clothes need folding, the bills need paying, but those things can and will get done, even if you take a little *you time* along the way. Maybe it means relaxing in a hot bath, indulging in your favorite dessert, or taking the day off. It can come in many forms, but always look inward to determine which needs aren't being met, and take some time for yourself.

Challenge of the Day: **Spend at least thirty minutes today (and each day) doing something for yourself. Read a book, take a hot bath, go for a walk; these are just a few ideas, but whatever it is, spoil yourself.**

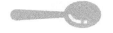

RECIPE OF THE DAY:

GREEN GODDESS SALAD

INGREDIENTS FOR GREEN GODDESS DRESSING ───────────

1 cup plain Greek yogurt
1 cup mixed herbs such as parsley and cilantro
1 avocado, chopped
1 ½ tablespoons chopped chives
2 tablespoons lime juice, plus ½ teaspoon zest
1 tablespoon extra virgin olive oil
1 teaspoon minced garlic
¼ teaspoon sea salt
Freshly ground black pepper

INSTRUCTIONS ──────────────────────

In a food processor, combine ingredients until well combined.
Season to taste.
Serve as a dip or toss with salad greens.

Dressing Serves 3-4
Prep: 20 mins
Cook: none

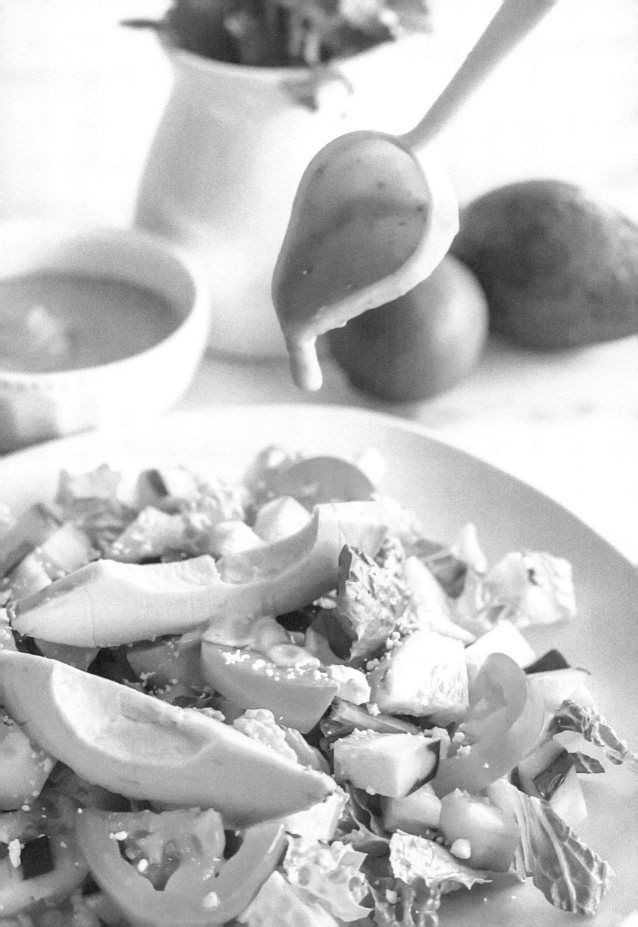

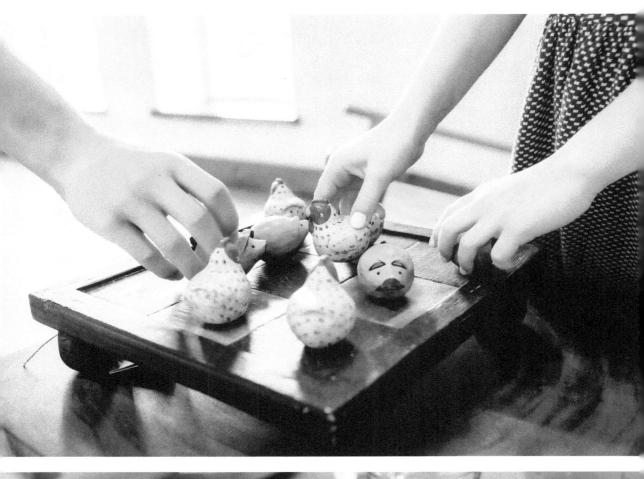

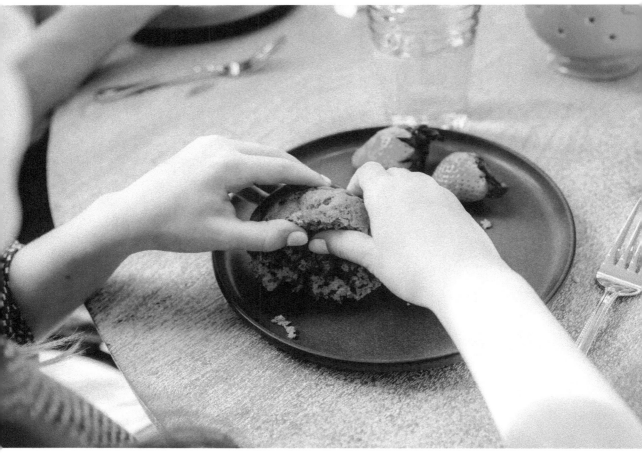

16
One Day at a Time

"The best thing about the future is that it comes one day at a time."
– Abraham Lincoln

A GLOBAL PANDEMIC IS NOT SOMETHING I EVER THOUGHT I would live through, and I imagine you can relate. This is probably why I spent so many hours watching, listening, and wondering what was going to happen next. Somewhere along the way, I began to realize how much I was being sucked into the negativity, and it was hurting more than helping. The good news is that when something big is happening in our lives, we only have to focus on the day in front of us. What do we need to do *today* to make it a good day? We are not going to solve the world's problems by lying awake all night, thinking about everything going on around us.

I can wholeheartedly relate to this in my life right now. We are in the process of moving and trading everything we know for the unknown. So many questions; How long will this process take? Will it be difficult to meet new people? How will the kids adjust? *One day at a time*—that's what I keep telling myself. I don't need all the answers right this very minute. We have a plan, and things may shift or change— but I trust that God has His hands on the steering wheel of my life and will guide me in the right direction. I rely on my faith to get me through the fears of the unknown.

Challenge of the Day: **Write down something you were worried about recently. Has anything changed about that situation? Take a deep breath and know that this too shall pass.**

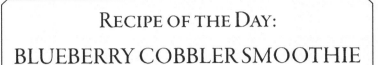

RECIPE OF THE DAY:

BLUEBERRY COBBLER SMOOTHIE

INGREDIENTS

1 cup frozen blueberries
1 frozen banana
¼ cup coconut milk
⅓ cup plain Greek yogurt
1 tablespoon honey
1 tablespoon granola
½ teaspoon freshly squeezed lemon juice
½ teaspoon cinnamon
A pinch of nutmeg

INSTRUCTIONS

Combine all ingredients in a blender and pour into glasses and serve.
Top with extra granola.

Serves 1-2
Prep: 5 mins
Cook: none

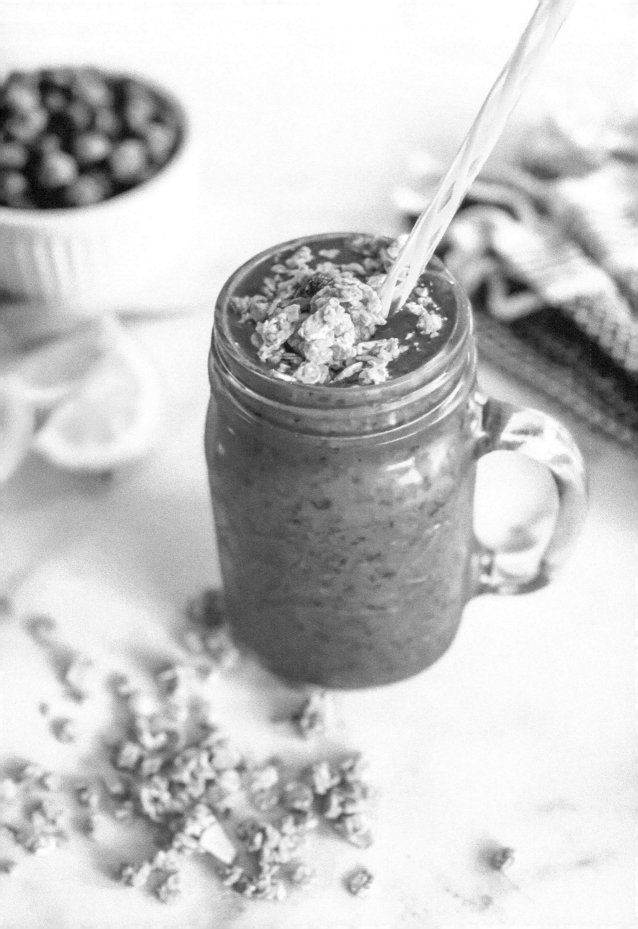

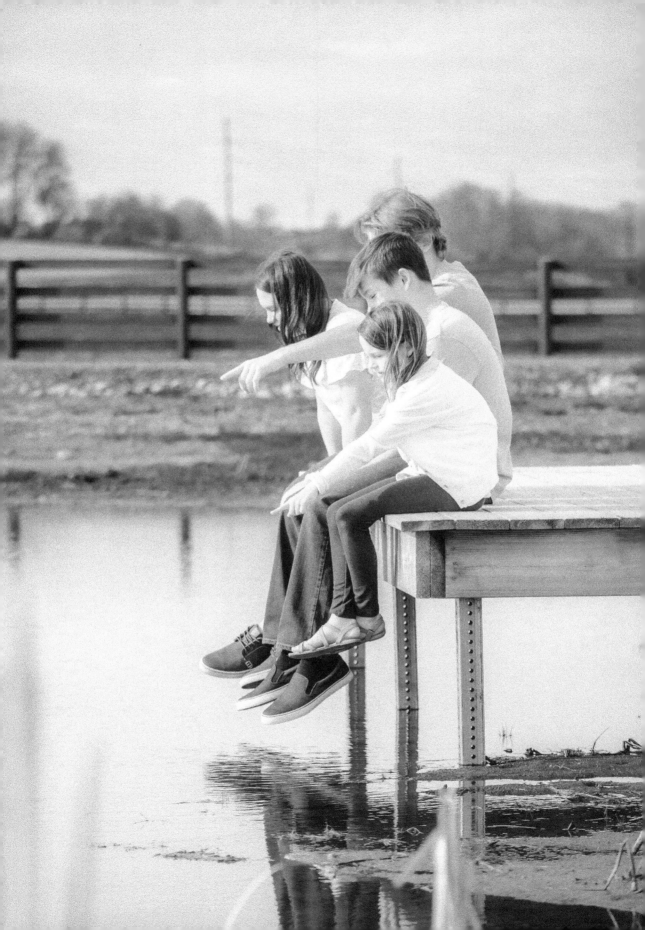

17

Explore

"If we were meant to stay in one place, we'd have roots instead of feet."
– Rachel Wolchin

NOT EVERYONE HAS THE LUXURY OF FANCY VACATIONS and traveling the world. But there is so much to explore right outside your back door! Even though I love Wisconsin, I often dread winter. However, after being stuck indoors for so long through the pandemic, I noticed something unusually beautiful about this past winter. The trees looked like a scene straight out from a *Frozen* movie—frost along every branch. It was breathtaking. How could I not have noticed this ever before?

The world around us is so full of beauty, it would be a shame for us never to enjoy it. When we find ways to get out and explore, we often find beauty in the most unexpected places.

Nature is amazing—the earth and rock formations, the way trees canopy over top hiking trails and butterflies soar in wide open fields. Spending time in nature can help clear your mind of worry and offer you the sense of peace you're longing for.

Challenge of the Day: **Search for a nearby hiking trail or walking path and spend an afternoon with nature.**

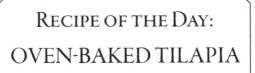

RECIPE OF THE DAY:
OVEN-BAKED TILAPIA

INGREDIENTS

4 tilapia fillets
½ lemon
1 ½ tablespoons melted butter

SEASONING

½ teaspoon paprika
1 tablespoon parsley
½ teaspoon garlic powder
Salt and pepper to taste

INSTRUCTIONS

Preheat oven to 400°F.
Rinse fillets, pat dry, and place on pan with cooking spray.
Drizzle with butter.
Squeeze lemon juice over fillets and add seasoning.
Cook 15 minutes or just until fish is flaky.
Broil for the last minute if desired.

Serves 4
Prep: 15 mins
Cook: 15 mins

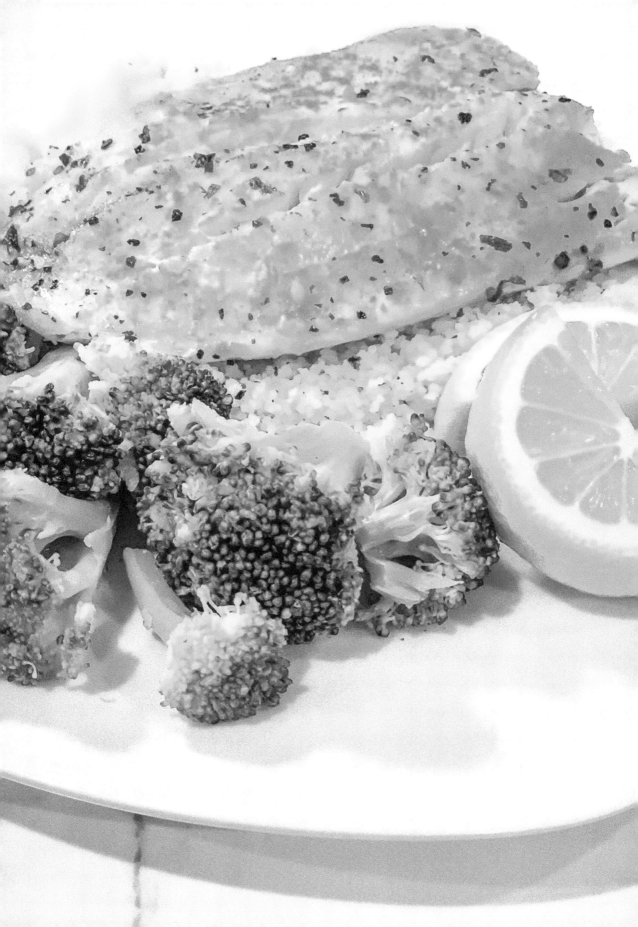

18
Forgiveness

"When you forgive you don't change the past, you change the future."
– Bernard Meltzer

WE'VE ALL BEEN WRONGED AT ONE POINT IN OUR LIVES. Someone offended or hurt us; someone deceived us. People make mistakes; that's what makes us human. We cannot hold on to every wrongdoing against us because it only hurts us in the end. Holding on to that kind of negativity will only interrupt the peace we desire in our lives.

No one can successfully drive a car forward while looking out the back window. In the same way, we cannot successfully move into the future while focusing on the past. We've got to let things go and continue on. That is not to say that forgiveness is easy.

The road to forgiveness is much like a roller coaster; there are many ups and downs that eventually lead to healing. Once we find peace within ourselves, we are able to move past the hurt and start again.

Forgiveness is not about accepting what happened, but knowing we deserve better. By forgiving those who hurt us we can open a new door that is free of pain and allow ourselves to move forward.

Challenge of the Day: **Life is too short to hang on to any kind of negativity. Forgive whomever you might need to forgive, even if that person is yourself, and move on.**

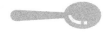

RECIPE OF THE DAY:
GREEN POWER SMOOTHIE

INGREDIENTS

1 cup fresh spinach
1 cup water
½ cup frozen mango chunks
½ cup frozen pineapple chunks
½ cup frozen avocado chunks
1 frozen banana, sliced
1 cup plain Greek yogurt

INSTRUCTIONS

Blend spinach and water about 40-45 seconds.
Add remaining ingredients and blend again.
Pour into glasses and enjoy.

Serves 1-2
Prep: 5 mins
Cook: none

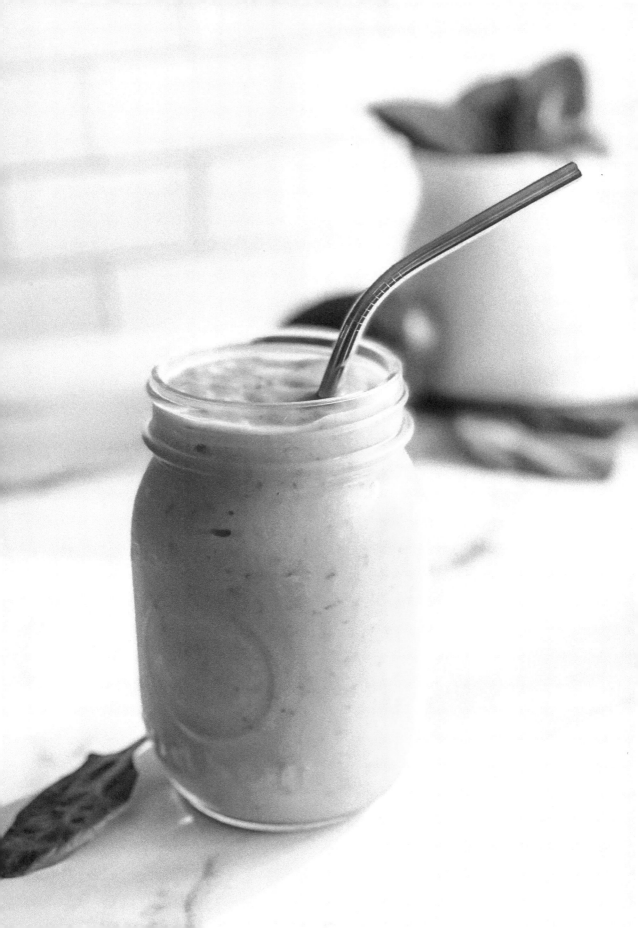

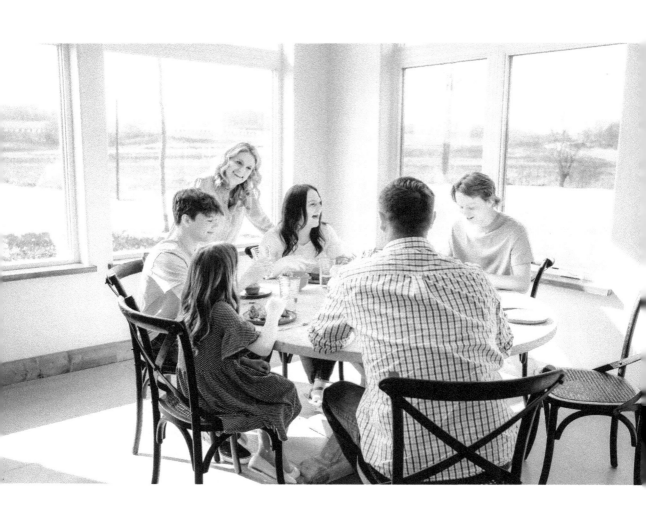

19
Laugh a Little

"A day without laughter is a day wasted." – Charlie Chaplin

WHO IS THE FUNNIEST PERSON YOU KNOW? I CAN TELL you mine (not in any particular order): my dad, my mom, my husband, my kids—oh, and me; it must run in the family...ha.

Laughter is the absolute best feeling in the world. And I promise you—it stays with you longer than you might think. I still feel joy in my heart from laughing with my dad thirty years ago. People ask me about him, and although my memories have somewhat faded, I very clearly remember how funny he was. I'm not sure if it was the way he spun everything into a joke or because he could lighten up any situation; he just made people laugh. I think he would be so happy to know that, after all these years, I still feel that joy. His jokes, his silly faces vividly remain in my mind and heart.

It makes me think—I want to leave something like that behind too; a little piece of joy long after I'm gone. Laugh a little. Find humor in situations and share it with people you care about.

Challenge of the Day: **Find a joke or a funny story that you can share with your family today around the dinner table. Maybe for dinner, try this recipe and ponder what a skinny chicken might look like.**

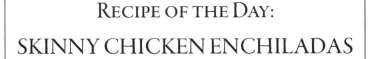

RECIPE OF THE DAY:

SKINNY CHICKEN ENCHILADAS

INGREDIENTS

2 cups cooked chicken breast
1 small yellow onion, finely diced
1 tablespoon garlic, minced
1 teaspoon olive oil
1 teaspoon cumin
1 teaspoon chili powder
1 can black beans, drained
½ cup verde salsa
1 (4 oz) can diced green chiles

1 ½ cup reduced-fat cheddar cheese
2 tablespoons butter
2 tablespoons all-purpose flour
1 ½ cup low-sodium chicken broth
1 cup plain non-fat Greek yogurt
Salt and pepper to taste
8 (6-inch) low-carb flour tortillas
¼ cup chopped cilantro
1 (2.2 oz) can sliced black olives

INSTRUCTIONS

Preheat oven to 375 degrees.
In a medium skillet saute garlic and onion with olive oil until soft.
Add chicken, cumin, chili powder, black beans, and salsa — stir and simmer on low 3-5 minutes.
Scoop mixture over tortillas, roll, and place fold-side down in a 9x13-inch lightly sprayed casserole dish. Set aside. Melt butter in a medium saucepan, add flour; stir frequently to create a paste.
Slowly stir in chicken broth, simmer about 3-5 minutes.
Add 1 cup cheese, ½ teaspoon cumin, green chiles, yogurt, salt, and pepper .
Stir until cheese is melted .Sauce will be slightly thin. Pour mixture over enchiladas, top with remaining cheese, and bake 30-35 min.

Serves 4
Prep: 20 mins
Cook: 30 mins

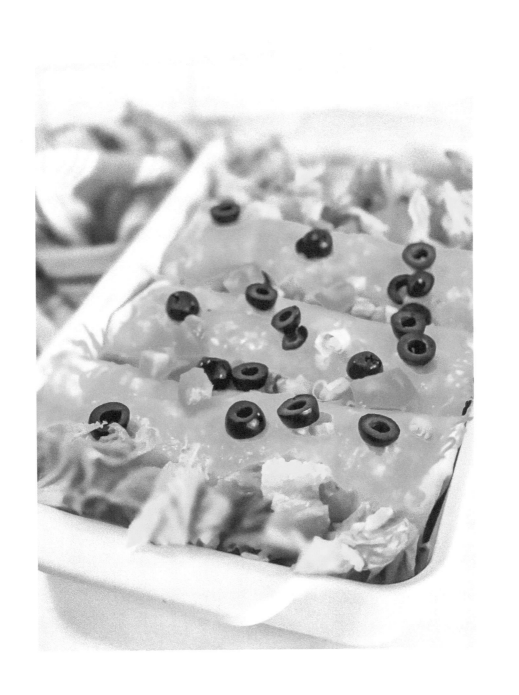

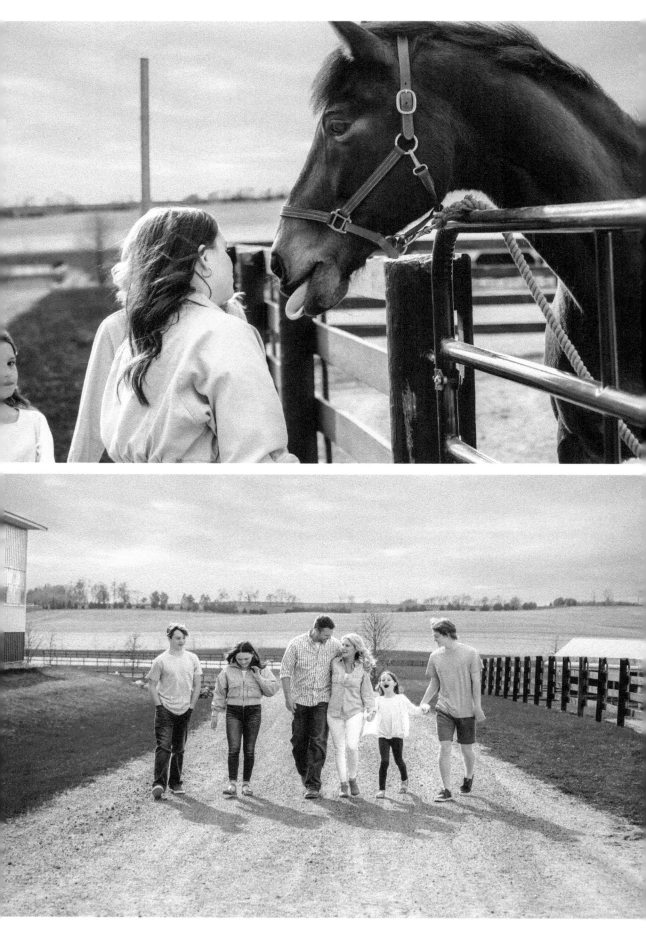

20
Don't Sweat the Small Stuff

"Remember, today is the tomorrow you worried about yesterday."
– Dale Carnegie

S IMILAR TO A FEW CHAPTERS BACK WHEN WE TALKED about taking things *one day at a time*, I want to dive a bit more into the *small stuff*, and how dwelling on these things can snowball and become huge burdens in our lives.

Those who know me will tell you, I shouldn't be writing a chapter on this. *I sweat the small stuff.* On the other hand, who better to tell you this than someone who can relate? Whatever keeps you awake at night, I'm with you. But then we wake up the next day and suddenly all the things we worried about hardly seem like anything at all. Certainly, there are things in life that warrant our concern, but at the end of the day, we have to come to terms with what we can and cannot control. Oftentimes, the *small stuff* fits into the "cannot control" category, so why worry?

I will admit, this is easier said than done. All too often I have focused too much on the details causing me to lose sight of the bigger picture. If I would have stepped away and not allowed myself to overthink, I could have saved myself many hours of lost sleep.

Next time you find yourself consumed with worry, I want you to come back to this page and highlight the quote above—*today is the tomorrow you worried about yesterday*. Don't sweat the small stuff.

Challenge of the Day: **Put a Post-it® note next to your bed that reads, "Do not worry about tomorrow; you already did that yesterday."**

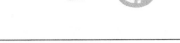

RECIPE OF THE DAY:

HEALTHY CHICKEN SALAD

INGREDIENTS

1 cup cooked and shredded chicken
1/3 cup light mayo
2 tablespoons Greek plain yogurt
1/3 cup red or green grapes, diced
½ green apple, finely diced
¼ cup celery, finely diced
Squeeze of lemon
¼ teaspoon black pepper
Pinch of salt

INSTRUCTIONS

In a large bowl, combine all ingredients. Serve on a romaine lettuce leaf or slice of bread.

Serves 2
Prep: 20 mins
Cook: none

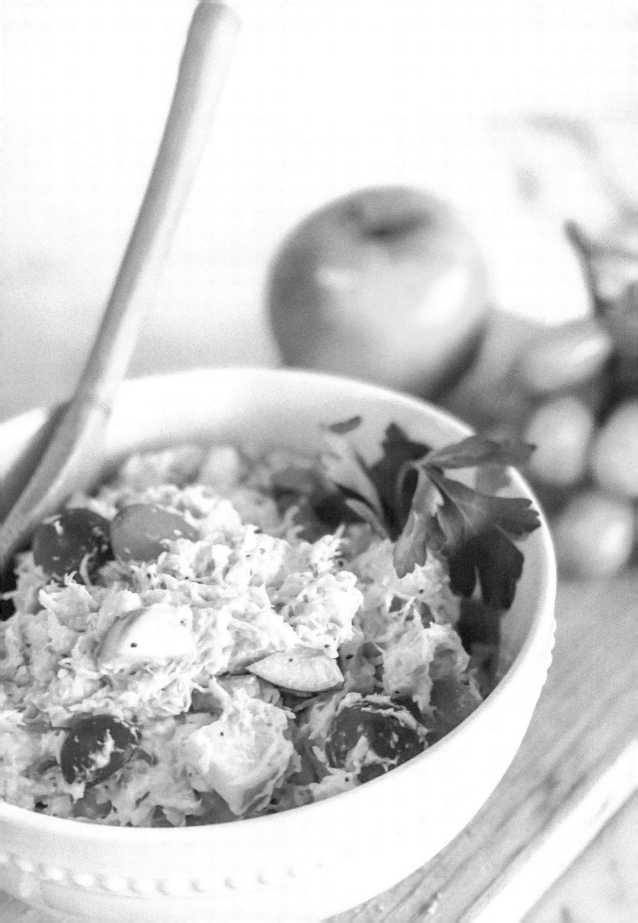

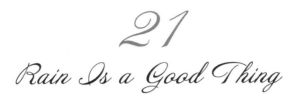

21
Rain Is a Good Thing

"Start washing all our worries down the drain, rain is a good thing."
– Luke Bryan

WHEN PEOPLE SEE RAIN IN THE FORECAST, THEY IMME-diately get discouraged. Rain ruins picnics, weddings, a fun day at the zoo... but have you ever thought about all the *good* rain can bring? Remember the farmer we talked about earlier in the book...and droughts? Without rain, we would not have fresh food and fresh beautiful flowers. Like the old saying "April showers bring May flowers," rain is a good thing.

The funny thing about rain is we like and appreciate it, but only on our terms. We want to be able to control when it happens. For example, I love the gentle sounds of rain on my window at night. But when I wake up in the morning, I want nothing but sunshine. Unfortunately, we don't get to pick and choose when the rain falls.

Rain shows up in various ways in our lives and not always in the form of drops. Rain can be an unplanned situation or unexpected event that catches us off guard. It could be losing a job or having to change schools. This kind of rain can leave us with disappointment and frustration.

When rain hits our lives and our plans have to be changed, we need to think of the bigger picture down the road. Maybe we'll understand it, maybe we won't ever— but know that not all rain is bad and recognize that it can actually be a good thing.

Challenge of the Day: **Think about *rain* you've recently had in your life that turned into something good. Let that be a reminder to you for future rainy days.**

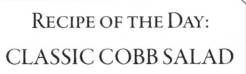

CLASSIC COBB SALAD

INGREDIENTS

1 bag (8 oz) mixed salad greens
2 slices of cooked bacon, crumbled
1 cup cooked and sliced chicken breast
1 hard-boiled egg, sliced
½ large avocado, sliced
1 Roma tomato, sliced
½ cup feta cheese, crumbled
1 cucumber, peeled & sliced

INSTRUCTIONS

Line ingredients over salad greens and serve with a low-calorie dressing of choice.

Serves 1-2
Prep: 20 mins
Cook: none

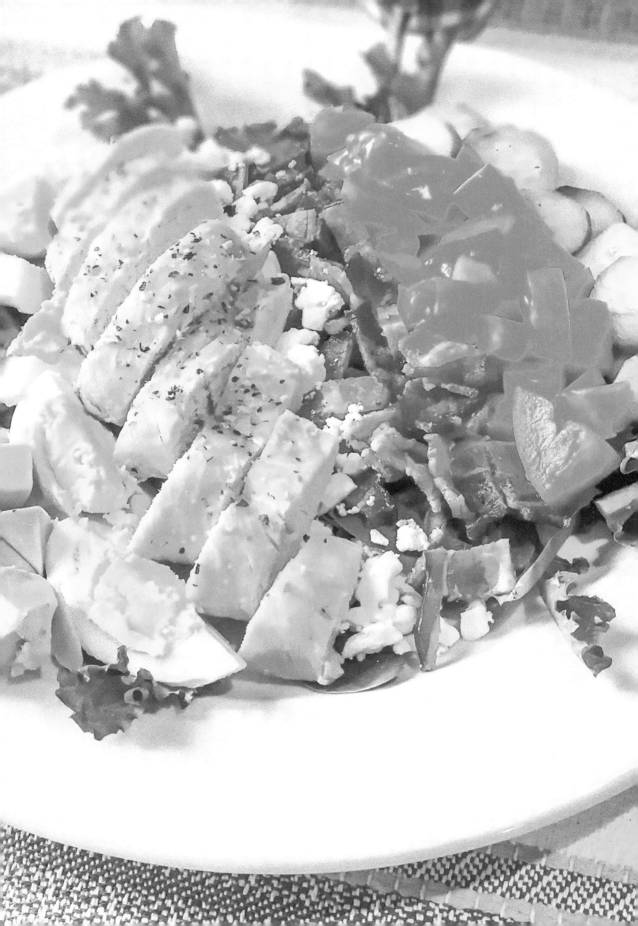

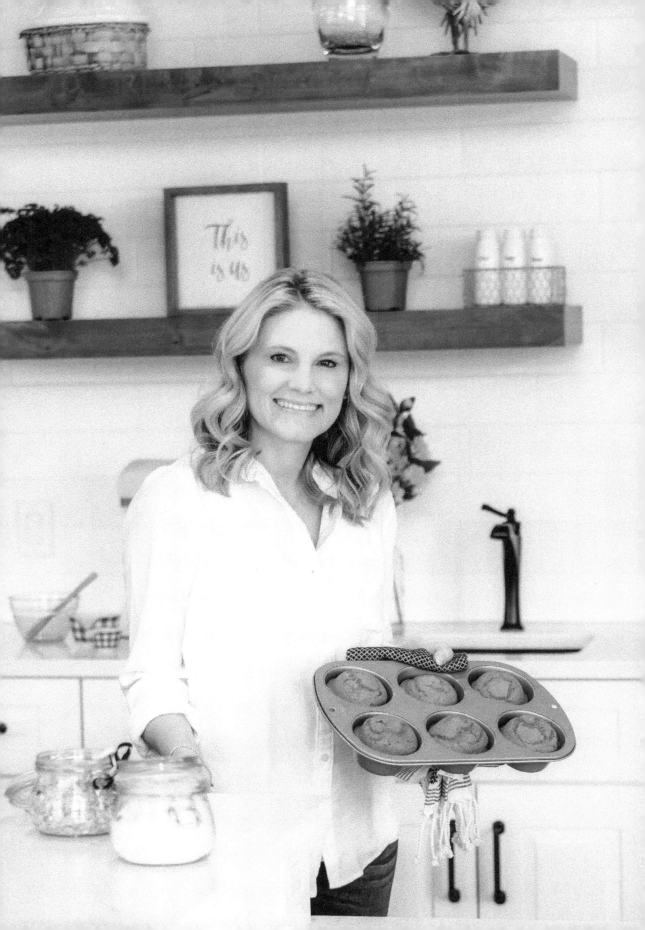

22
Smile

"A smile is the prettiest thing you can wear." – Ali Edwards

IN THE TELEMARKETING WORLD, EMPLOYEES AT CALL CEN-
ters are often trained to "respond with a smile." This may seem silly since tele-
marketers are not interacting face to face with their customers at all. There is a lot
of power in a smile. The simple act of smiling can turn your day around, boost your
mood, and enhance your immune system. A smile is free—it costs nothing. It takes
only a second but can last forever in the hearts of those who receive it. A smile cre-
ates healthy relationships at home and at work and is uniquely owned by YOU.

Think back to moments when you were shopping and the difference in your experiences between dealing with a frowning employee behind the cash register and
the one who was grinning from ear to ear. Which one would you be more likely to
return to?

Just the simple act of smiling can have such a meaningful impact on the lives of those
who see it. Remember this when you're feeling like there's nothing you can do to
change the world around you. Challenge yourself to change it one smile at a time.

Challenge of the Day: **Take a picture of your smile and send it to a friend, post
it on social media, or simply print it out for yourself to keep.**

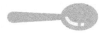

Recipe of the Day:

SKINNY BUFFALO DIP

INGREDIENTS

3 cups cooked and shredded chicken
1 cup Frank's Red Hot Sauce
2 (8oz) packages Neufchâtel cheese, softened
1 cup plain Greek yogurt
½ packet ranch seasoning
1 cup shredded reduced-fat cheddar cheese, divided

INSTRUCTIONS

Combine shredded chicken and buffalo sauce in a pan over medium heat.
Mix cream cheese, yogurt, and ranch dressing in pan. Stir in cheddar cheese
until melted.
Once everything is melted and combined, place mixture in a medium sized
casserole dish. Top with remaining cheese and place in the oven for 15 minutes at 450 degrees.
Serve with your choice of vegetables, crackers, or pita bread.

Serves 4-6
Prep: 20 mins
Cook: 15 mins

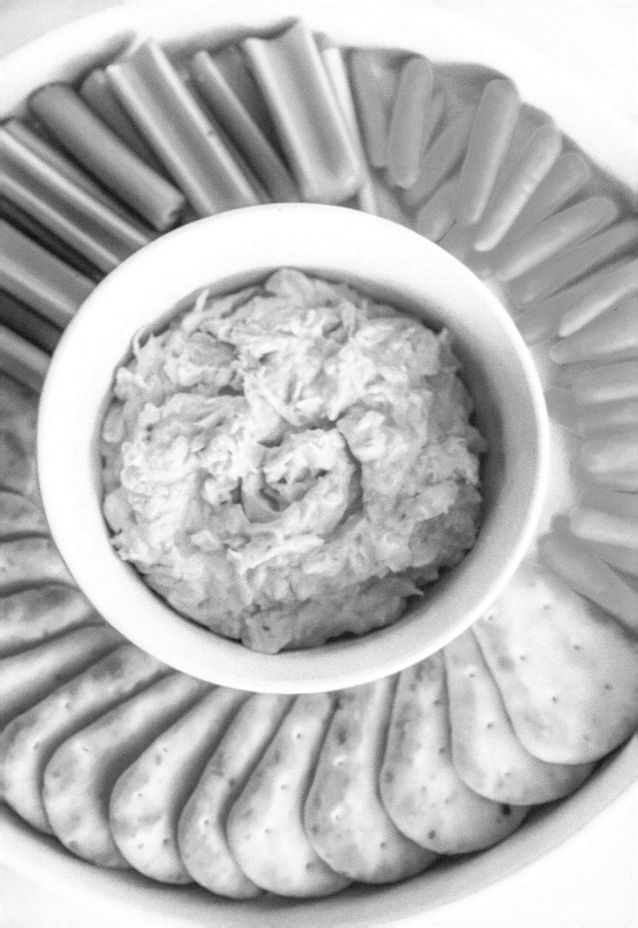

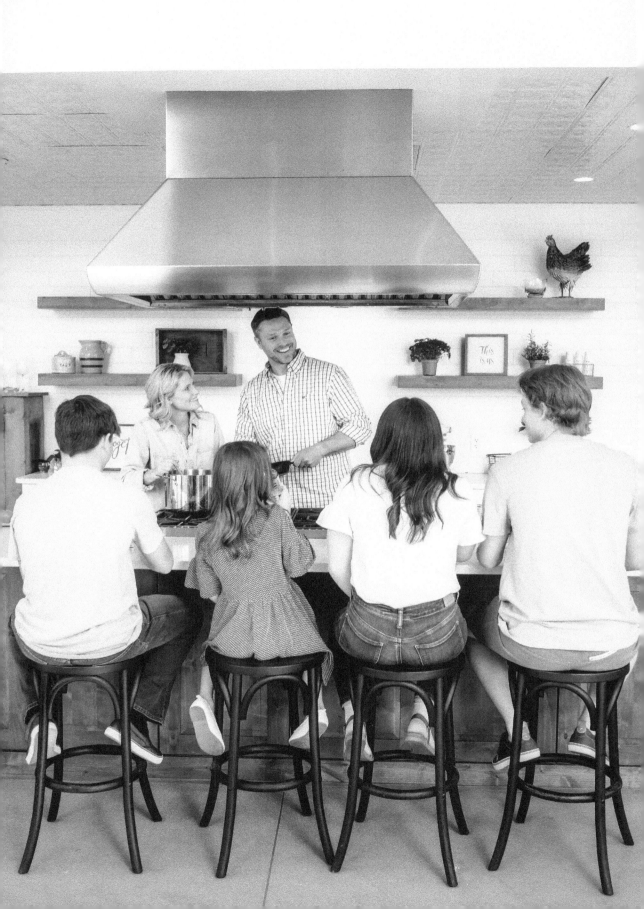

23
Secret Ingredients

"The secret ingredient is always love." – Unknown

WRITING A COOKBOOK IS LIKE TELLING THE WORLD ALL your best-kept secrets. I like developing my own recipes, but sometimes I enjoy making old family-favorite's that have been handed down to me. Those recipes are a little harder to get my hands on—No one likes giving up their *secret ingredients.*

Have you ever gotten a recipe from a relative, followed it exactly, only to find that it just didn't taste the same? Sometimes that is because it is missing the *secret ingredient*—the person who gave it to you. It could be the difference in the butter they chose or the way they mixed their ingredients by hand instead of using a mixer. Whatever the case may be, sometimes even if a recipe is followed exactly, it tastes different.

Recipes can turn out great whether they are followed exactly or with a few new or extra ingredients.

Same goes in life. There are many ways to find joy and happiness, but none of them include one "secret" ingredient that makes everything perfect. Sometimes a hug will be just what we need, and other times a quiet night with family does the trick. Life is never perfect. We each have to discover what works for us because in life...*we* are the secret ingredients! Each of us bring our own flavor to the world around us. If we don't like something, we can change it, we can try a new ingredient. Eventually we will have a recipe for happiness that is just right for each of us.

Challenge of the Day: **Take a recipe that you always use and try adding a new ingredient to the mix.**

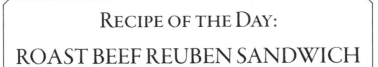

ROAST BEEF REUBEN SANDWICH

INGREDIENTS

1 (8oz. can) sauerkraut, drained
⅓ cup low-fat mayo
3 tablespoons sweet and tangy mustard
1 pound roast beef deli meat slices
1 package baby swiss cheese slices
Loaf of seedless marbled rye bread

INSTRUCTIONS

In a small saucepan, combine sauerkraut, mayo, and mustard; simmer on low and stir frequently.
Fold slices of deli meat in half and place on a flat, heated skillet. Layer multiple slices to preference. Turn with spatula. Place swiss cheese over deli meat until melted. Toast rye bread in toaster oven. Remove deli meat from skillet and place on one slice of toasted rye bread. Spoon sauerkraut mixture over cheese and top with toasted rye bread.

Serves 2-4
Prep: 15 mins
Cook: 10 mins

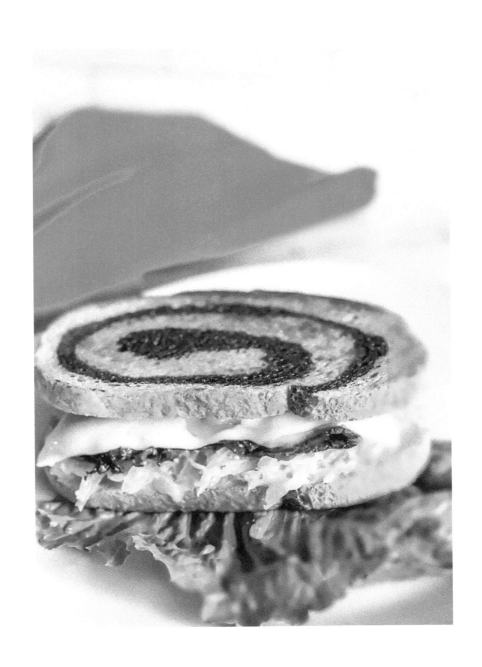

24
Mistakes and Endurance

"I don't think there's any chef that is born great like in music or in sports. You have to burn yourself...messing up makes you a better chef." – David Chang

I've been told that in the English heritage, families were often named by their profession. Since my maiden name is Baker, it must mean someone along my bloodline was a baker, which I find a little bit ironic since I don't really like the act of baking. It's not that I can't bake, it's more about the *process* that baking involves. The whole act of exact measuring throws me off; I'd much rather toss in a few spices and herbs.

So, if I'm going to be honest, my biggest issue with baking is actually the small margin for error. Add a little too much water and your cake can go flat. Add a little too much flour and it can be dry. There's not much room for error, and I'm not too keen on mistakes in the kitchen.

Learning and growing are all part of the process. Whether you are trying to be a better chef, athlete, business owner, farmer, parent, student, or whatever else you might have your sights set on, remember this—you will make mistakes. Learn from them and continue forward—set goals and achieve them. Why? Because you can. If we shy away from every challenge, nothing new or exciting would ever come about.

Challenge of the Day: **Try baking these muffins. If I can do it, so can you.**

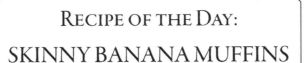

RECIPE OF THE DAY:

SKINNY BANANA MUFFINS

INGREDIENTS

2 ripe bananas
1 cup unsweetened applesauce
1 large egg
1 tablespoon vanilla extract
3 tablespoons brown sugar (Swerve)
2 tablespoons coconut sugar
1 teaspoon ground cinnamon
1 teaspoon baking powder
½ teaspoon salt
1 ½ cups all-purpose flour
2 tablespoons unsalted butter, melted

INSTRUCTIONS

Grease large muffin pan.
Preheat oven to 350 degrees.
Mash bananas in mixing bowl.
Combine egg, applesauce, vanilla, brown sugar, coconut sugar, and cinnamon.
Stir well to combine. In a separate bowl, stir together flour, baking powder,
baking soda, and salt. Add flour mixture to banana mixture. Combine and add
butter; do not over-mix.
Spoon batter into muffin pan and bake for 18-20 minutes.

Serves 6 large or 12 regular-size muffins
Prep: 15 mins
Cook: 20 mins

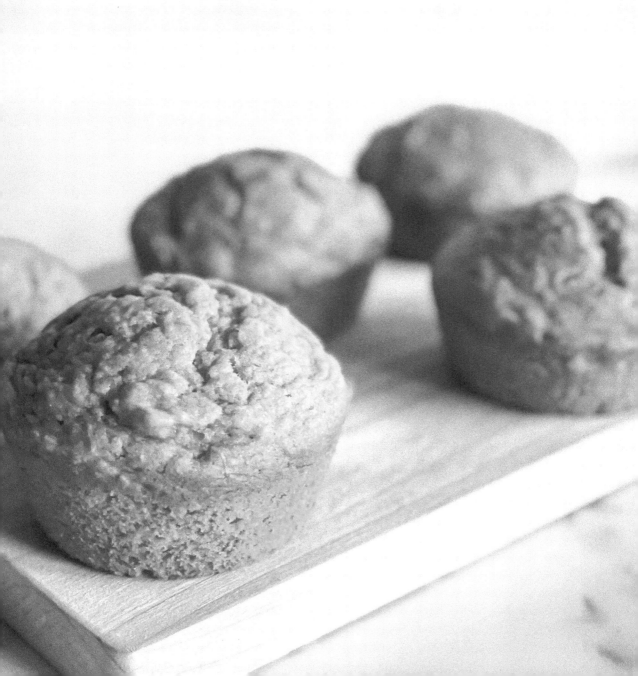

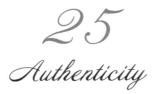

25
Authenticity

"Life is too short for fake butter or fake people." – Julie Child

WE TALKED ABOUT STAYING TRUE TO WHO YOU ARE AND pushing through obstacles that are in your way. I also want to take a moment to talk about authenticity. Authenticity is aligning your core values and beliefs with your actions. When I stop to think about this word, I realize how all the other topics in this book help lead us toward being our authentic selves.

People will always have different opinions, values, and beliefs than us; this doesn't make them more wrong or right, just different. Over time, I have gotten more comfortable with letting go and just being me. Conforming to what others think and their collective thoughts and opinions does not allow me to be authentic. Likely, we've all encountered this at some point in our lives.

It is our individuality that makes the world a beautiful place. If everybody was a teacher, who would take care of the sick? If everybody was a farmer, who would fix our cars? The list of professions are endless. The world needs me just as I am, and it needs you just as you are. Our authenticity adds different flavors to the mix.

Be mindful of this as you go about your days. Stay true to who you are—because YOU are awesome and your values and opinions matter.

Challenge of the Day: **List three people in your life who are authentic, true friends. Call them, message them, or text them today to let them know you value them.**

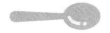

RECIPE OF THE DAY:
BALSAMIC PEAR SALAD

INGREDIENTS

1 bag (8 Oz) mixed salad greens
2 pears firm but ripe, thinly sliced
½ cup dried cherries
½ cup feta cheese, crumbled
½ cup candied pecans, chopped

INSTRUCTIONS

Place all items together over salad greens and drizzle with Balsamic dressing of choice.

Serves 2
Prep: 15 mins
Cook: none

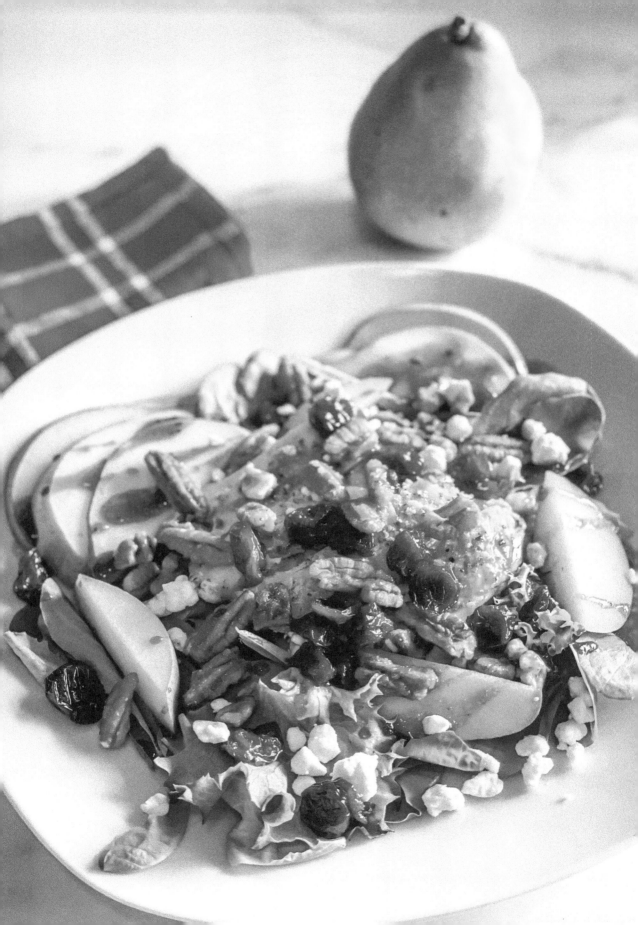

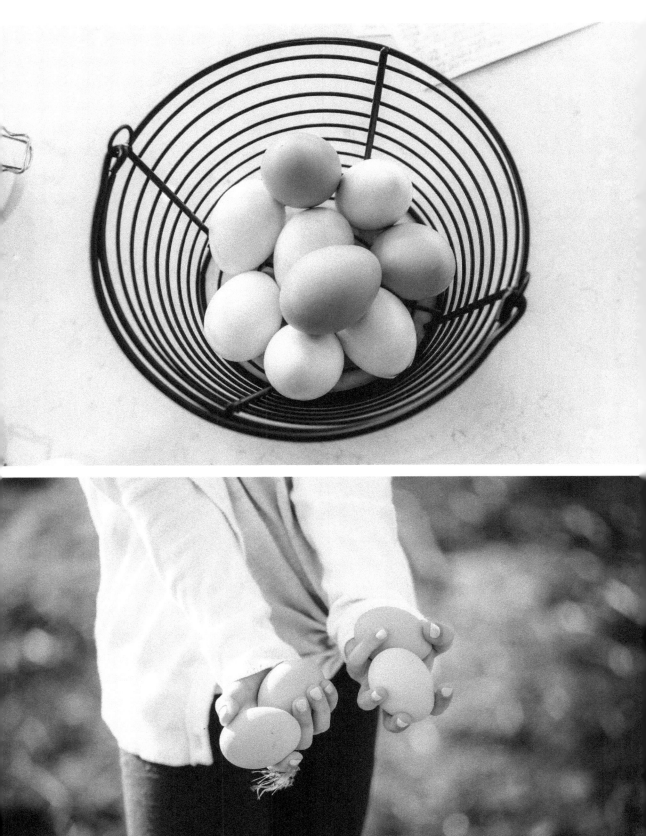

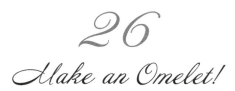

26
Make an Omelet!

"I think pressure's healthy and very few can handle it." –Gordan Ramsey

Most of us have heard the phrase "When life gives you lemons, make lemonade." Well, as you know we have chickens so instead we say: "When life cracks your eggs, make an omelet."

Life doesn't just give us sour moments; sometimes it breaks our plans altogether. The pandemic was a prime example of this. So many people had plans for 2020. They thought they knew how their job would look, their vacation, their shopping experience, but suddenly everything turned upside down. When an egg is cracked, it no longer looks the same. The same is true for whatever plans we might have. When our plans get cracked, they no longer look the same—but that is not necessarily a bad thing.

In times like this, we learn to be resourceful. Oftentimes, people never really know what they are capable of until their comfort zone has been broken or stripped away. I'm not saying we would choose a pandemic, but we sure can look back and see what all the amazing people around the world have done to get us to where we are today.

Chances are you can think of a time when something discouraged you to the point of cracking, but yet here you are still standing. Proof that you can be resourceful—you made your omelet.

Challenge of the Day: **Crack an egg and make a real omelet! If you need some inspiration, use the recipe of the day.**

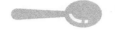

RECIPE OF THE DAY:

VEGETABLE OMELET

INGREDIENTS

4 large eggs
Olive oil cooking spray
¼ cup chopped broccoli
¼ cup chopped onions
¼ cup diced tomatoes
¼ cup finely diced carrot
¼ cup shredded cheddar
Salt and pepper to taste
Fresh parsley

INSTRUCTIONS

Whisk eggs in a small bowl with salt and pepper. Heat a medium skillet sprayed with cooking spray. Poor egg mixture into pan. Add vegetables across egg mixture. Sprinkle with cheese, fold over, and serve.

Serves 4
Prep: 15 mins
Cook: 30 mins

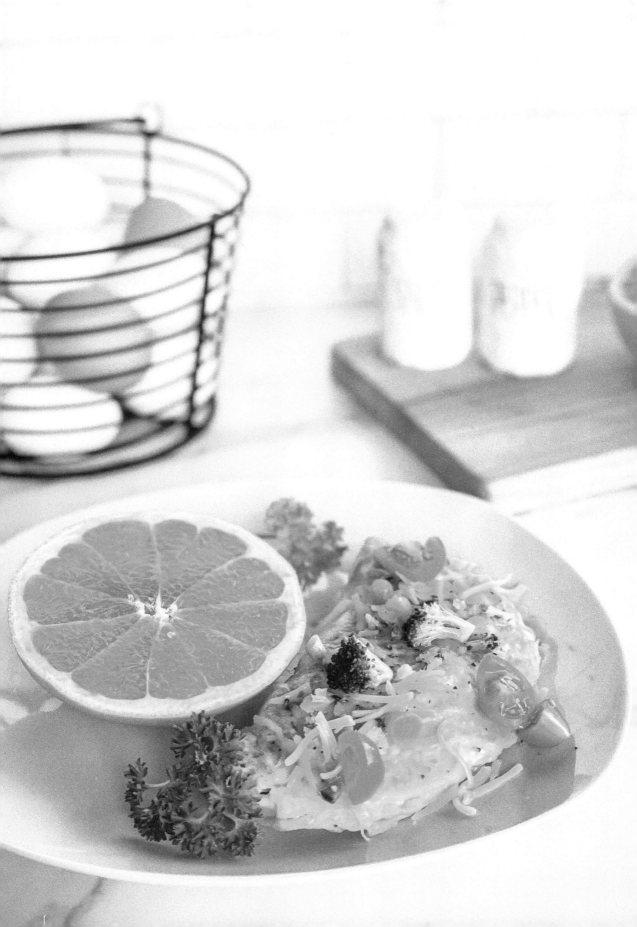

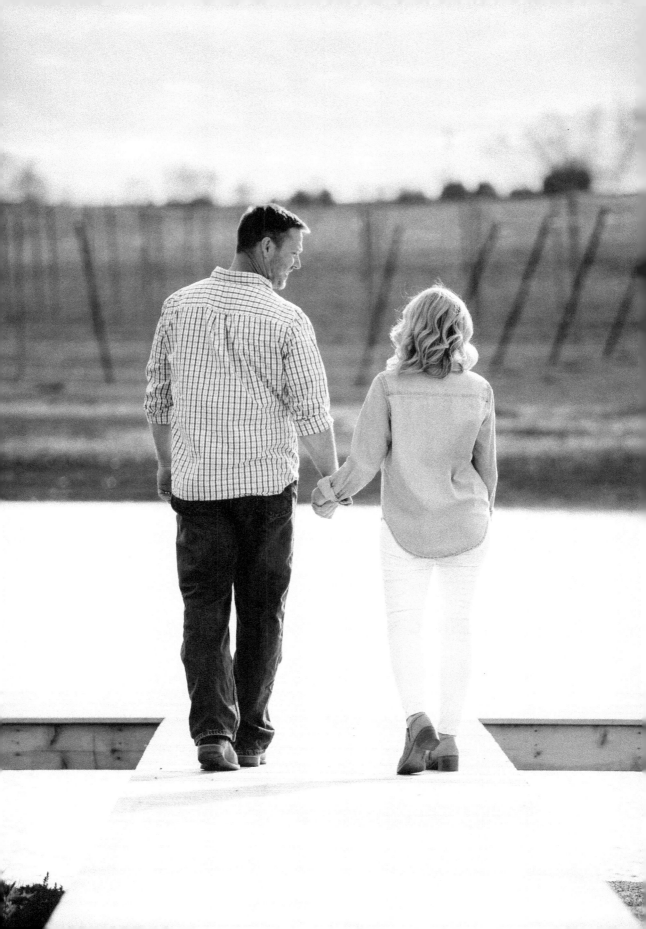

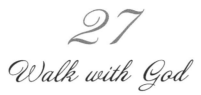

27
Walk with God

"The lord is near to all who call on him. To all who call on him in truth."
Psalm 145:18 (NIV)

I BECAME A CHRIST FOLLOWER AFTER MY FATHER PASSED away thirty years ago. I had always gone to church prior and was raised in a Christian family, but this was when my real walk with God started. I started attending church regularly and was baptized a few months later. My relationship with God most definitely carried me through that difficult time; and still does to this day.

Having said that, there have been times in my life when I felt closer to God than others. My walk with Him has not always been steady. Just like any relationship, ours with God is no different. When we take time to commit and put forth effort into our faith, we walk with God and see the calmness and beauty that exists within it. It is easy to get distracted and find ourselves more distant when we don't make our relationship with God a priority in our lives.

Throughout my blog and while writing this book, I have felt God's presence more than ever. I know that I am right where I am supposed to be. I am always learning how to grow more in my faith—and will continue my spiritual growth as I remain committed to my walk with God.

Challenge of the Day: **Take a moment to find a Bible verse that resonates with you. Write it in the back of this book with a permanent marker.**

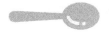

RECIPE OF THE DAY:

IMMUNITY BOOST SMOOTHIE

INGREDIENTS

½ cup freshly squeezed orange juice
1 cup peach or vanilla Greek yogurt
½ frozen banana
¼ cup unsweetened almond milk
1 cup ice
½ teaspoon ginger paste

INSTRUCTIONS

Combine all ingredients together in a blender until smooth.

Serves 1-2
Prep: 5 mins
Cook: none

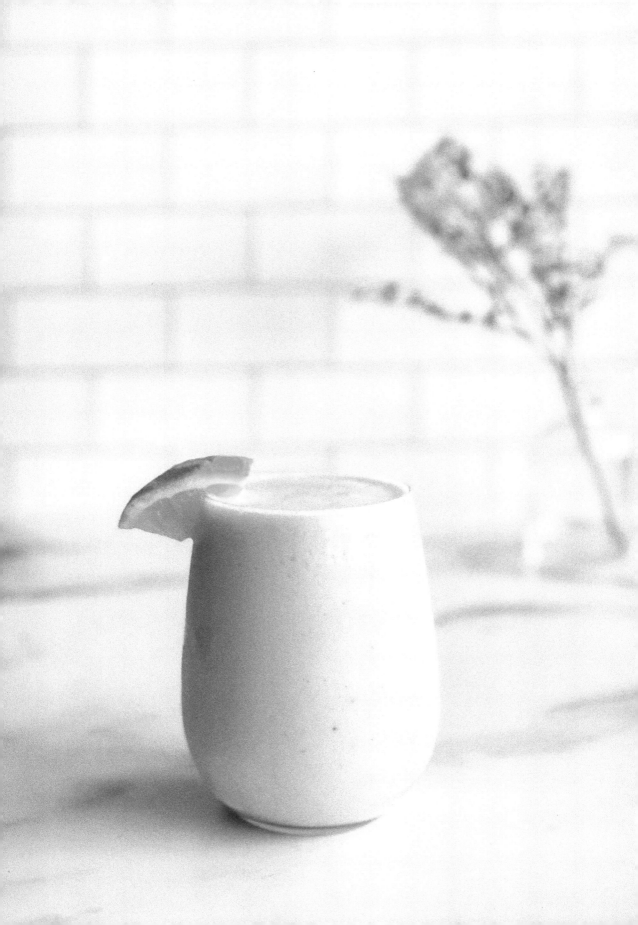

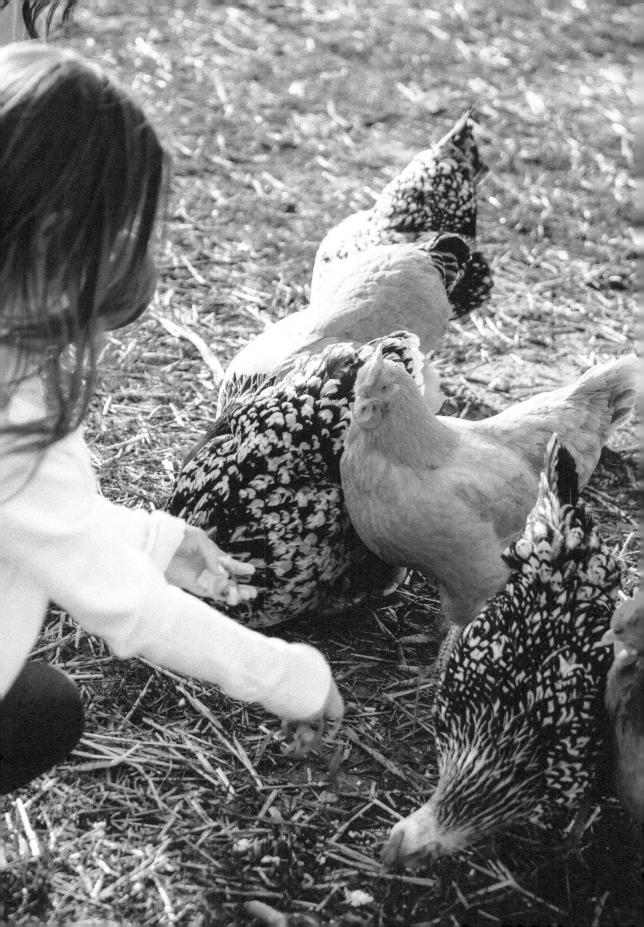

28
Be the Change

"You never know what people are going through, and sometimes the people with the biggest smiles are struggling the most, so be kind." – Unknown

EACH DAY ON MY BLOG, I START WITH A POSITIVE QUOTE or Bible verse similar to the structure of this book. I do this in hopes that it will encourage someone to pay it forward or be extra kind to a stranger that day. I do it because maybe the person reading it is going through a difficult time. All too often we are blinded to the struggles others face, and we don't consider the outcome of our actions.

As I mentioned early on, I lost my father when I was young. He was a kind and gentle soul who loved me deeply, but silently struggled with depression. My desire to inspire kindness and positivity is in hope that we can be the change the world needs for people like my dad and those who face unseen hardships and challenges.

It doesn't take much for us to do our part. If each and every one of us made a little effort to be more understanding and have more compassion, we could really change the world we live in and be the strength to those who need it most.

When I pick out a positive quote or scripture, it is often one that speaks to me that day. Oftentimes, it is easy for us to forget that everyone around us is human too. Even if they look like they have it all together, they still have moments where they struggle with doubts and uncertainties. For this reason, we all must strive to be the change we want to see in the world around us.

Challenge of the Day: **Be conscious of your thoughts, actions, and words. Do one random act of kindness today—this can be as simple as texting an old friend, complimenting a coworker, or sharing positive words on social media.**

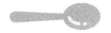

RECIPE OF THE DAY:
TILAPIA FISH TACOS

INGREDIENTS

2 tilapia fillets
¼ teaspoon paprika
¼ teaspoon garlic powder
¼ teaspoon cumin
Salt and pepper to taste
4-6 low-carb flour tortillas

PINEAPPLE SLAW

2 cups shredded cabbage
¼ cup light mayo
1 lime, juiced
¼ teaspoon salt
1 teaspoon apple cider vinegar
¼ cup fresh pineapple chunks
Cilantro, chopped

INSTRUCTIONS

In a small bowl, combine cabbage, mayo, lime juice, pineapple, cilantro, vinegar, and salt. Chill until ready to serve.

In a separate bowl, mix garlic powder, paprika, cumin, salt, and pepper. Season each tilapia fillet on both sides. Preheat oven to 400 degrees. Place tilapia fillets on a baking sheet with cooking spray; bake for 10-12 minutes or until fish is white and flakey. Slice fish into pieces and lay over a spoonful of slaw on a low-carb tortilla. Garnish with pineapple, lime, and cilantro.

Serves 2
Prep: 15 mins
Cook: 15 mins

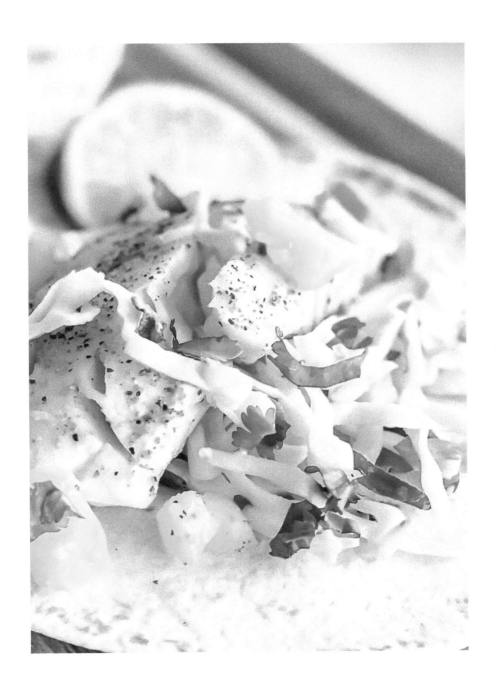

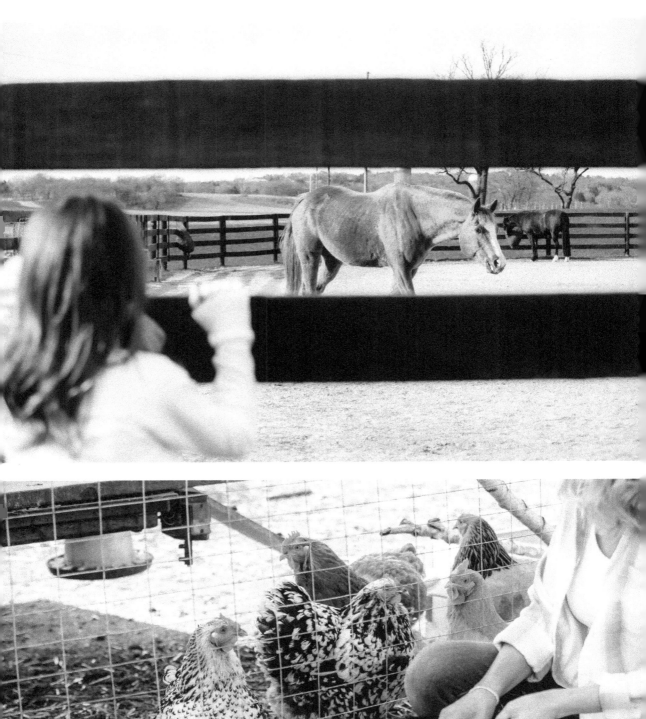
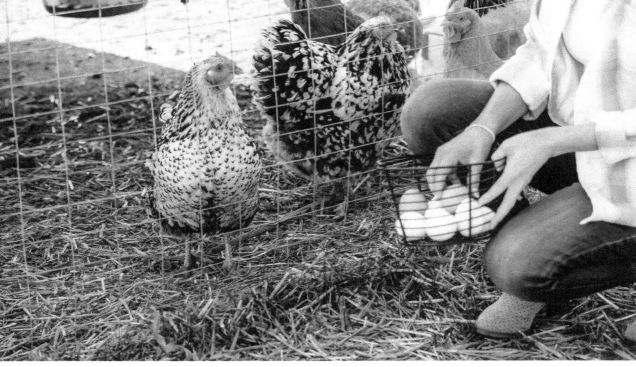

29
Don't Stop Believing

"Some will win, some will lose, some were born to sing the blues."
– Jonathon Cain

THE BAND JOURNEY KNEW WHAT THEY WERE DOING WHEN they wrote this song. Not only would it be the number-one karaoke song in the world (which I know all too well from years of hogging the microphone), but this song would inspire so many people with the words, "Don't stop believing." It is something, for whatever reason, we must hear over and over. No matter how far we go, there will always be an unknown that seems a bit scarier than the last one we crossed. The history behind the lyrics of this song is worth noting. Jonathon Cain, who eventually joined the band Journey, was unemployed and discouraged the moment he heard the words of his father over the phone saying, "Don't stop believing."[17] He jotted those words down in a notebook, without a clue that it would later become one of the most famous songs of all time.

We must remember where we have been and what we have gone through in our lives. Doubt, worry, fear—these things will always crash into us and prevent us from keeping our cups full to the brim. Life is worth exploring, growing and thriving, not just surviving. The less we plan to do, the less we *will* do.

All that we've talked about over the previous pages of the book has been a gathering of ingredients for this wonderful dish called life. It is worth living! With gratitude, passion, and forgiveness, it is worth stepping outside of our comfort zones and taking chances here and there. When we implement these things in our own lives, it is easier for us to encourage others and say, "Don't stop believing."

Challenge of the Day: **Make a list of five things you want to do this year. Then, make it happen!**

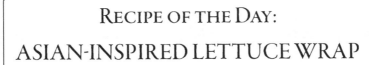

RECIPE OF THE DAY:

ASIAN-INSPIRED LETTUCE WRAP

INGREDIENTS

1 pound ground turkey
1/3 cup carrots, finely diced
1/3 cup onion, finely diced
1/3 cup celery, finely diced
2 tablespoons olive oil
Lettuce leaves (butter or romaine)
Green onions, finely sliced
Salt and pepper to taste

SAUCE

2 tablespoons Hoisin sauce
1-2 tablespoons Sriracha sauce
3 tablespoons coconut aminos or low-sodium soy sauce
1.5 tablespoons rice vinegar
3 tablespoons brown sugar (Swerve)
2 tablespoons sesame oil

INSTRUCTIONS

In a medium skillet, heat olive oil and add carrots, onions, and celery. Sauté until softened and onion is translucent. Add ground turkey; season with salt and pepper to brown. Cook until no longer pink. In a small bowl, combine sauce ingredients; add sauce to ground turkey and vegetables. Stir and simmer on low.
Serve over lettuce leaves.
Top with diced green onions and sesame seeds.

Serves 3-4
Prep: 15 mins
Cook: 20 mins

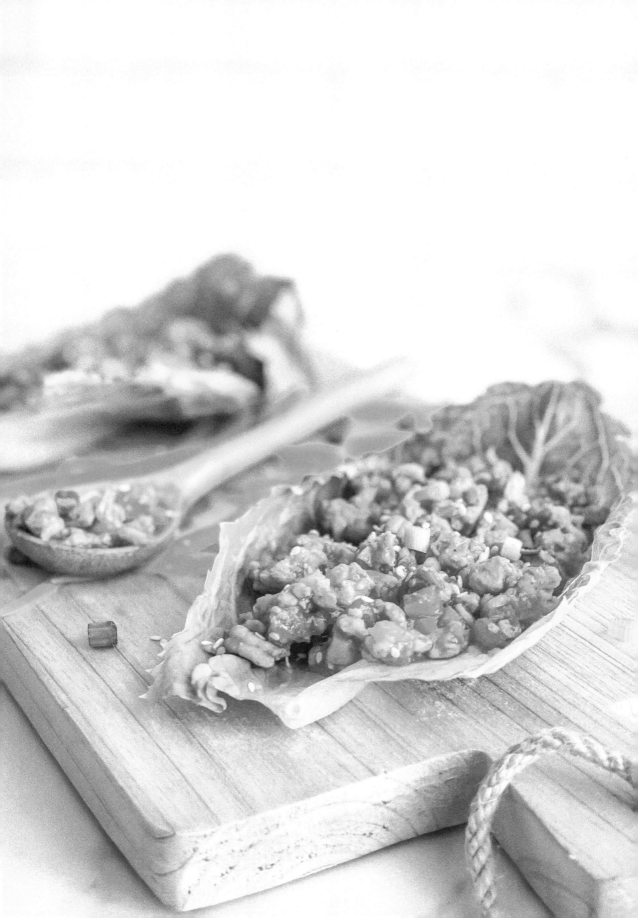

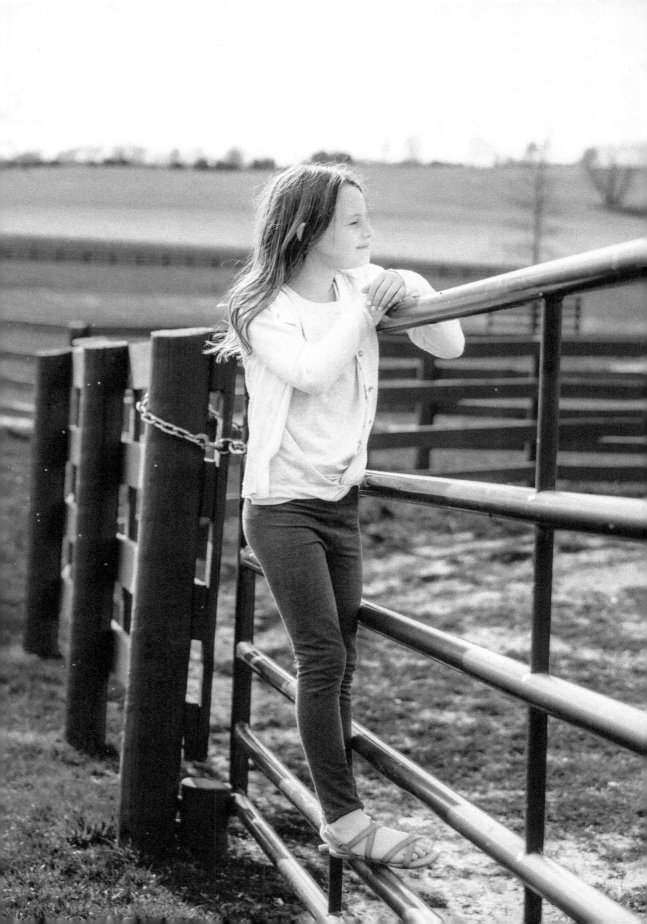

30
New Perspective

"Every day is a new beginning, take a deep breath, smile and start again."
– Ain Eineziz

LIFE IS A JOURNEY.

We get out of it what we put into it. We make choices along the way—who will join us and who will we depart from? Who will we learn from and who will we teach? Where will we spend our time and where will we not? This book has come into existence through my own journey—through the choices I've made along the way of what I would and would not let hold me back.

I'm thankful and grateful to have been given this opportunity to invite you into my kitchen. I hope the messages you've heard have inspired you to—dream big, love deeply, explore, cherish others, try new things, and, most importantly, live your best life. I hope you've found a recipe or two you can enjoy along the way.

Challenge of the Day: **Write down five things you are going to take from this book and implement in your life. Look forward to a fresh, new day with a fresh, new outlook.**

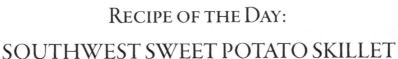

RECIPE OF THE DAY:

SOUTHWEST SWEET POTATO SKILLET

INGREDIENTS

1 teaspoon olive oil
1 pound lean ground beef
½ small yellow onion, diced
2 teaspoons chili powder
2 teaspoons cumin
1 tablespoon minced garlic
2 cups cubed sweet potatoes, cooked
1 can diced tomatoes
1 can seasoned black or chili beans
1/3 cup shredded Monterey Jack cheese
2 tablespoons Tabasco Green Pepper Sauce
Cilantro for garnish
Salt and pepper to taste

INSTRUCTIONS

In a large skillet, heat olive oil over medium heat. Add onion, garlic, and ground beef.
Brown until crumbled.
Add chili powder, cumin, salt, and pepper.
Simmer 1-2 minutes, stirring frequently.
Drain meat; remove excess grease from skillet.
Add sweet potato, tomatoes, beans, and Tabasco sauce.
Stir and simmer while covered 5-7 minutes.
Serve in a bowl topped with cheese and fresh cilantro.

Serves 4
Prep: 5 mins
Cook: 15 minutes

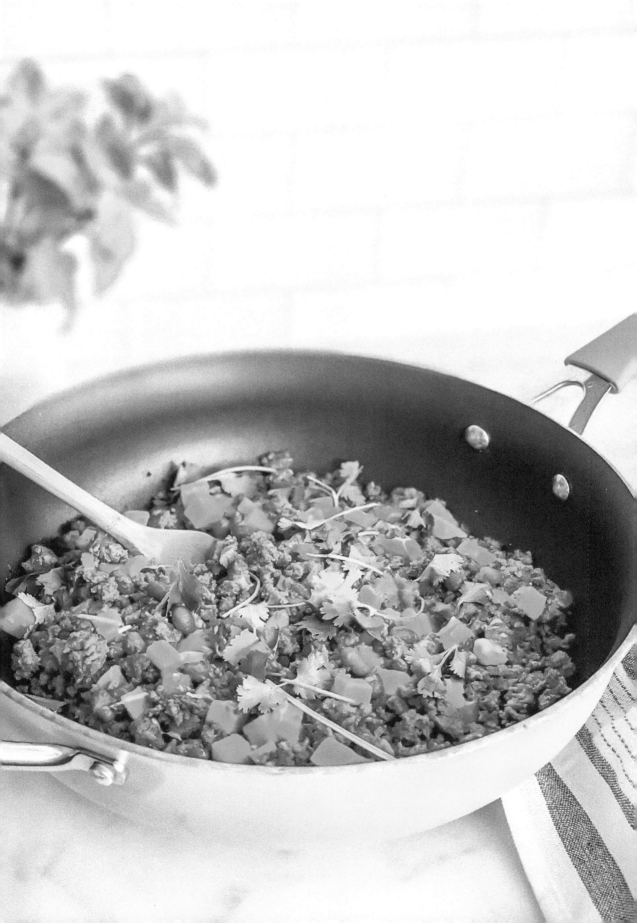

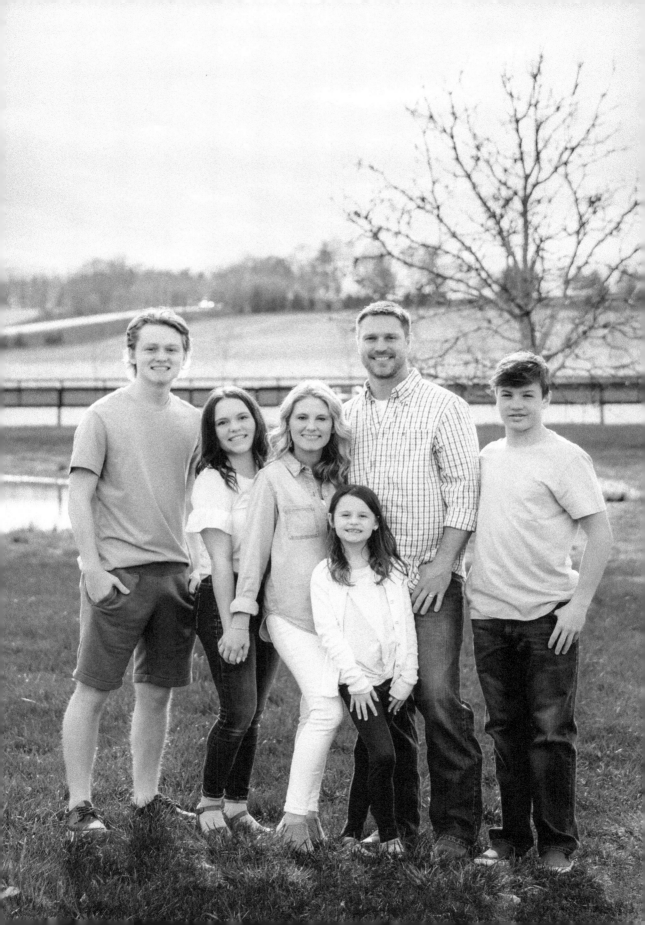

Notes

Notes

Notes

Notes

Endnotes

1   https://plantbasedlowcarb.com/coconut-flour-vs-all-purpose-flour-a-viable-substitute/

2   https://www.verywellfit.com/monk-fruit-benefits-side-effects-uses-4588601

3   https://www.healthline.com/nutrition/liquid-aminos-benefits#:~:text=What%20Are%20Liquid%20Aminos%2C%20and%20Can%20They%20Benefit,hunger.%206%20Easy%20to%20add%20to%20your%20diet

4   Why Almond Flour Is Better Than Most Other Flours (healthline.com)

5   https://plantbasedlowcarb.com/coconut-flour-vs-all-purpose-flour-a-viable-substitute/

6   https://www.healthline.com/nutrition/natural-sugar-substitutes#69.-Natural-sweeteners

7   https://www.healthline.com/nutrition/natural-sugar-substitutes#69.-Natural-sweeteners

8   https://www.healthline.com/nutrition/natural-sugar-substitutes#69.-Natural-sweeteners

9   How to Substitute Applesauce for Sugar (healthfully.com)

10 The 7 Best Substitutes for Sour Cream (healthline.com)

11 Why and How to Use Coconut Oil to Replace Butter? | MD-Health.com (md-health.com)

12 Neufchâtel Cheese vs Cream Cheese – Differences, Calories, Fat, Carbs (yourhealthremedy.com)

13 Quotescover.com

14 https://greatergood.berkeley.edu/article/item/why_gratitude_is_good

15

16 https://lenwilson.us/5-thing-geese-can-teach-us-about-teamwork/

17 https://americansongwriter.com/dont-stop-believin-journey-behind-the-song/

Lightning Source UK Ltd.
Milton Keynes UK
UKHW051249100821
388547UK00003B/24